TO SEND A DOVE

One Woman's
Triumph over Breast Cancer

Delores Hackett Rutherford

Mayhaven Publishing

Mayhaven Publishing
P O Box 557
Mahomet, IL 61853
USA

Cover Art © Patrick Jordan

Cover Design by Cullen J. Porter

Copyright © 2000 Rutherford

First Edition—First Printing 2000
1 2 3 4 5 6 7 8 9 10
LOC: 00 41115
ISBN 1-878044-79-6

To Marie,

May this book be a blessing to you.

Delores Hackett Rutherford

This book is dedicated to the memory of:

Robert J. Hackett, my loving husband

Lowell W. Woodall, my loving father

Joy Deliece Crouse, my loving sister

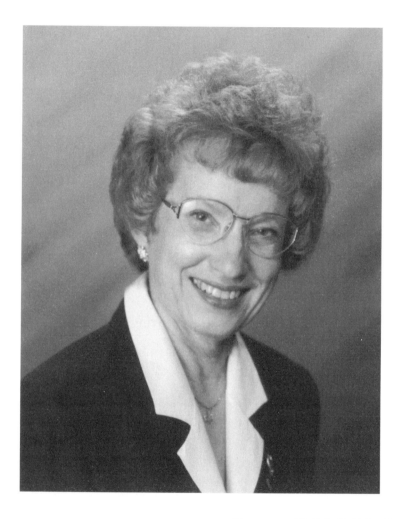

Delores Woodall Hackett Rutherford.

Acknowledgements

Thirteen years have passed since the first fledgling lines of this book were penned. The journey to completion has been long and arduous, and without the encouragement of others, I'd have given up long ago.

Most supportive was Bob Hackett, my husband and partner of nearly 35 years. Knowing his desire for this book equaled mine gave me courage to keep working after he was gone from my life.

Members of the National League of American Pen Women, Quad Cities Branch, offered invaluable critique. "Cut it in half," they instructed. Thank you, Connie, Karen, Jeannie, Dee and Barb.

To my children, Diana, Tammy and Terry and their spouses, Kurt, Gary and Anne, I say: Thanks for saying the work was good when it wasn't, and for helping me keep the dream alive.

Thanks to Carolyn, whose gift of a porcelain dove reminded me that she believed, too. Thank you, Sandy, for your frequent offers of homemade cookies for the first book signing.

Finally, my heartfelt thanks goes to my husband of three years, Jim Rutherford, for his desire to share this adventure in faith with me. After great losses in our lives, we now walk together in newness and love.

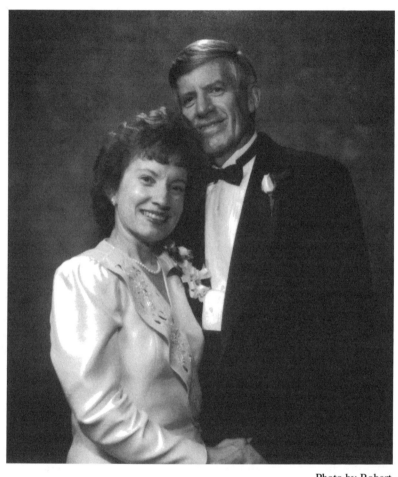

Photo by Robert

Bob and Delores Hackett, August, 1991.

Contents

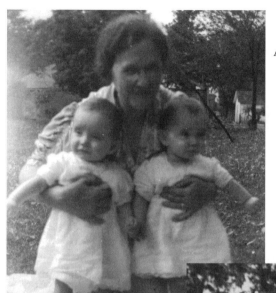

At left: Grandma Nora Ann with me, Jane Delores (left) and my twin, Joy Deliece.

At right: Deliece (right) and I dressed for our high-school prom. Similar in many ways, both of us would experience cancer.

Introduction

The statistics hit me like a blast of cold air on a January morning.

"According to figures released by the American Cancer Society," Dan Rather of CBS's 48 Hours reported, "one hundred seventy-five thousand new cases of breast cancer will be diagnosed this year, 1991. More than 44,000 women will die as a result of this disease."

Staggering numbers, I thought.

"One out of three women with breast cancer will die," he continued.

I was tempted to turn off the program. I'd heard enough gloom and doom about breast cancer. The topic seemed to be a favorite of every news-magazine and talk-show host on television. I reached for the "remote," poised to make this grim news disappear. But, the hour was late and I was tired. With little energy to do anything else, I watched the report.

"Breast cancer is a disease on the attack; breast cancer attacks older women; those who smoke; those who eat too much fat and too little fruit and fiber; those who exercise too seldom; those who have a family history of cancer." *The dis-*

ease, I thought, *also assaults women whose bodies are specimens of good health.*

Any woman, it seemed, had the potential to become a victim of breast cancer.

Today, nine years later, the news for all women who fear breast cancer is more promising. Every day, women are cured from this dreaded disease. True, the incidence of breast cancer has risen to a projected 182, 800 new cases in the year 2000, but the percentage of those who survive has also increased from 66% to 78%.

Women today, however, remain as frightened of breast cancer as they were in 1991. Newspaper columnists, television news anchors and talk show hosts report of "women in crisis" because of breast cancer. These women search for a message of hope. Can anyone bring this message to them?

Yes. I can.

More than thirteen years have passed since I underwent a modified radical mastectomy. Cancerous lymph nodes forced me to undergo seven months of chemotherapy. Yet I am alive and healthy today. In thirteen years, cancer hasn't re-occurred. I embrace life fully—travel, enjoy grandchildren, praise God for each wondrous day.

Once cancer entered my vocabulary, I became nearly obsessed to share my experience. Women and their families need to know there is proven reason to maintain hope in the fight against breast cancer. Women also need to know that the love of God is the greatest healer of all.

Within these pages I share my innermost feelings, with the hope that my struggles and eventual conquests will encourage others engaged in personal battles, cancer and otherwise, of their own.

Some days with cancer were difficult. More often, though, my story is one of joy—joy of family and friends, joy of God's grace, joy of physical and spiritual healing. When our spirits lagged, God sent a dove of peace to encourage my husband and me.

No two women will experience breast cancer exactly alike; each woman's collision with this disease is hers alone. Even so, I am certain many aspects of my encounter with breast cancer will be appreciated by those facing similar struggles.

May this book bring hope to all who read it.

Delores Hackett Rutherford

Delores Hackett Rutherford

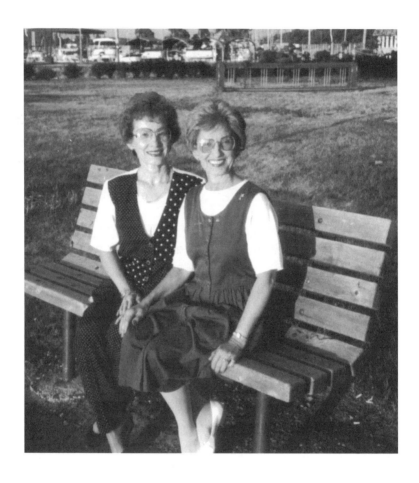

With my sister, Deliece, sharing one of our many pleasant moments together. Over time, our roles would alter, depending on the circumstances and our personal skills or limitations.

A Little Lump

"Peace I leave with you, my peace I give to you"

John 14:27

Surely this was a bad dream. Or maybe my lab report had accidentally been switched with someone else's. I'd heard of situations where that had happened. It seemed obvious there had been a serious mistake. This was too horrible to be true.

I kicked off my shoes and stretched out on the living-room couch to sort out my thoughts. Deep breaths helped calm my racing pulse. Through the window, the afternoon sun filtered softly through the sheers. The room was so quiet I could hear the ticking of the clock in the kitchen around the corner.

Everything had happened so fast. Nothing made any sense. I closed my eyes to the light, hoping to erase the incredible images that flashed in my mind. Instead, I began to replay each unforgettable scene in my head. Slowly, carefully, minute by unbelievable minute. *Oh, God, please help me.*

* * * * * * * * *

The whole thing had begun with a little lump. No big deal, I thought, whenever I remembered to investigate the tiny knot hidden beneath the slightly sagging muscle and tissue that formed my left breast. I'd learned to live with the lump, with no more regard for it than the mole beneath my nose or the vaccination scar on my shoulder. It was just there—obscure and unobtrusive—a minor thing in my fast-paced life. When I pressed my fingers against the lump, I was reminded of the eraser tip of a pencil. After each of the two mammograms since the lump's discovery eighteen months before, my doctor assured me it was the non-worrying kind, so I hadn't even prayed about it, and I prayed about many things—in the shower and the car, during solitary walks and quiet times, early in the morning and late at night. But I never prayed about the lump. It seemed so inconsequential—small and firm to my touch, but never painful or the least bit bothersome. When I fingered it to be sure it hadn't disappeared or grown larger, it seemed the same, so I was satisfied. At any rate, I was as healthy as a plate of alfalfa sprouts. There wasn't any reason to worry about the lump.

I might have dismissed it even further if it weren't for the urinary-tract infection that forced me to call my internist, Dr. Spivey. "What a bother," I muttered as I drove the few minutes across town to his office. A cold February wind whipped at me as I hurried inside the door. I tried to remember the last time I'd seen him. Probably for my yearly Pap smear.

I shivered on the examining table with a paper blanket around me, trying to keep warm. It was embarrassing to sit there undressed, but I smiled and pretended this was my favorite pose. "Good afternoon," the doctor said, flipping through my chart. He was a small man, about forty years old, I guessed. From the look of his disheveled hair, wrinkled lab coat and crooked tie, it appeared he'd had a busy day. When I thought about it, he had looked like this the last time I saw him. "Hello, Doctor," I replied.

Dr. Spivey examined me, then scanned the pages of my chart, again. Since the discovery of the lump in my breast, I'd suspected my records contained a reminder in big red letters— Always Check Lump!

He closed the folder and looked evenly at me. "We should schedule you for another mammogram," he said. "Your last one was in July." I must have been right about the chart.

Regular mammograms were important, I knew. I couldn't reasonably object. Besides, the previous experiences were swift, the way I liked them, and relatively painless. I nodded in agreement. "Whatever you say."

Days later, I registered at the Regional Breast Center in one of the local hospitals. The waiting area was attractive with its mauve and pink decor. Green plants and almost-current magazines were placed throughout the room.

"Hospitals are a lot more inviting these days," I said to the nursing attendant.

"We try," she said with a warm smile as she led me around the corner to a tiny room. I donned a pink gown, then followed her across the hall where an elaborate, ten-foot machine stood in the center of the room. I leaned stiffly against it, shivering at

15

the touch of cold metal.

The nurse kneaded and pulled my breast between plexiglass paddles that jutted out from the apparatus like vice clamps on my father's workbench. I winced as she increased the pressure on my flattened breast. Her fingers were bony and frigid. I drew back, sucking in my breath.

"Sorry," she said. "I know this is uncomfortable."

"Have you ever thought of putting a space heater in here?" I said dryly as I awkwardly embraced the machine, noting the goose bumps that decorated my arms. My lame attempt at humor did little to warm me or relieve the pain of my squished breast.

She grinned. "No, but maybe we should." I watched her slip a large screen into slots at the back of the machine, then quick-step around the corner.

Click. Click. I stood unmoving, pinned between the plates like a hapless butterfly. I'd be relieved to have this process over and prove my fitness to those who were concerned.

The nurse returned, released me from my restraints and turned me around to pummel the other breast.

"You may get dressed now," she said after the second x-ray. "Your doctor will notify you of the results."

I was grateful to return to the warmth of the tiny dressing room. In the long mirror on the wall, I studied my reflection. I could never determine whether I was pretty, but my father thought I was. So did my husband, Bob. He always tried to make people feel good, though, so his opinion was considerably weighted.

Mother had seldom been satisfied with my appearance, especially the size of my waist and the style of my hair. Consequently, most of my adult life I'd been obsessed with staying thin and having attractive hair. God's special blessing to me was a gift of natural curls and Mother's warm smile. These attributes had been sufficient to secure my twin sister, Deliece, and me positions of status in our small-town high school.

The farm and small town had long since been left behind in favor of the Iowa-Illinois Quad-cities (Davenport, Bettendorf, Rock Island and Moline), a community of more than 250,000 or so that hugged the Mississippi River. The metropolitan area offered arts, culture, sports and theatre without losing its sense of rural living.

I posed in front of the mirror, satisfied with the slight increase in weight from my size 10 wedding weight nearly 30 years before. My short, brown hair was neatly coifed. *Not bad for a 49-year-old mother of three.* I might not know much about my insides, but my outer self seemed acceptable.

I waved to the receptionist on my way out. "See you next year."

* * * * * * * * *

Dr. Spivey's call to my desk in the Athletic Office at Moline High School surprised me. I strained to hear the internist's quiet voice over the clatter of students in the hall. Did he say I should meet with a surgeon to discuss a biopsy? Surely there was nothing to be concerned about. How could

there be a problem? I'd never encountered any pain or dis-
charge, and the mammograms of the past had both appeared
good. I reached instinctively under my jacket. The lump felt
the same as always. My heartbeat, however, was racing.

"I'll arrange an appointment with a surgeon next week,"
Dr. Spivey said.

"Okay. I'm sure I can adjust my schedule."

I hung up the phone. Why did he call me at the office? Was
this urgent, or did he call all his patients at their work numbers?
Maybe he did. Maybe the call meant nothing. It was probably
easier to reach people at their jobs. Yes, that made sense. The
call was surely routine. There was no need to worry about it.

* * * * * * * * * *

I hurried home from the office to wash my face and brush
my teeth before my appointment with the surgeon. It was
important to make a good impression when we met.

At the bedroom door, I paused to admire the woodwork I'd
sanded, stained and varnished when the ranch-style home was
built eleven years earlier. *Good job*, I thought. Despite raising
three kids, the woodwork still looked new.

This house was tremendously important to me. Sided in
natural wood stained brown, with brick across the front, all the
exterior trim also bore my brush strokes. Maybe it was my
physical investment in the house that fostered my strong
attachment to it. Bob and I had dedicated the home to God

soon after we moved in.

I stood in the bedroom, gazing through the window toward two giant oaks behind the house. Their enormous branches spread across the lawn like canopies over a garden party. It was a joy to sit on the deck in the summer and watch squirrels chase through the branches and down the great tree trunks. Sometimes, brilliant cardinals sailed by, pausing momentarily on the huge limbs to serenade each other and me.

Now, with the trees bare, I could see houses on the opposite side of the ravine behind our lawn.

The view through the window today was peaceful. But how peaceful would my world be after my appointment with the surgeon? Grim memories of Mother, Grandma and Bob's mother unraveled my tranquility. Cancer had claimed each of their lives. Until now, though, I had blissfully ignored the possibility of cancer attacking me. With a healthy, happy life, my calendar crowded with activity, why would I want to think about cancer?

I stood quietly in the bedroom doorway. Maybe it was time to think about it now. Maybe I'd been a fool to ignore the truth all this time. Maybe this little lump finally deserved some prayer.

It was a few short steps to the queen-sized bed Bob and I shared. I sank to my knees, my fingers silently folding together. My head fell against the bedspread.

"Lord," I whispered, "this could be a big day. Please be with me."

* * * * * * * * * *

19

"Hello, Delores," Dr. Douglas said.

He's so tall, I thought, stretching to look into his face. At least six foot five, and as thin as he was long.

"Hello, Doctor." I reached to shake his hand. His dark-rimmed glasses, thick, gray hair and moustache accented an easy smile and made him look distinguished.

He motioned toward the examining table. "Please sit down." I hoisted myself onto the padded table and glanced around the small, gleaming room. Everything in it was white enamel or stainless steel.

Dr. Douglas eased his lanky body onto a round stool, rolled it against the wall and leaned his head back. Neither of us spoke while he studied the papers and charts I'd brought from Dr. Spivey.

Without looking up, he said suddenly, "One out of every nine women develops breast cancer."

My breath caught in my throat. "That's a high percentage," I stammered.

I came here to find out I'm okay, not talk about cancer. How can those numbers be possible? I know only a few women with breast cancer, and all of them are years older than me. Is this man trying to frighten me? I gulped air and searched the face of the surgeon. My initial kind appraisal of him now hovered on the brink of labeling him "enemy."

Dr. Douglas rose from the stool and walked toward me. "Let's see about this lump," he said lightly. "You'll need to undress to the waist."

I removed my blouse and bra and dropped them on a nearby chair, then eased back to lie down on the table. Dr. Douglas moved to my side and began pressing my breasts with his fingers.

"I can feel the lump," he said.

"Yes, that's the spot." I avoided looking at his face. The room was so quiet I could hear his breathing.

"All right," he said, "you may get dressed."

I searched his face for some clue to his thoughts.

"I feel you should have a biopsy," he said at last.

The breath went out of me and I jerked as though he'd thumped my knee with a padded hammer. My shoulders felt as though they were bound with tape.

"You've caught me off guard," I said weakly. "I thought you'd say everything is fine and send me home humming a tune."

"I know," Dr. Douglas said. A trace of a smile crossed his face. "But I think a biopsy is best. We need to be sure about these things." I watched his solemn face and dark-rimmed glasses as he returned to the low, round stool. Even with his back turned, he seemed to be watching me, too.

He's right about the biopsy, I thought. Six months earlier, at my last mammogram, the x-ray nurse made a comment that caused me to anticipate a biopsy, but Dr. Spivey had assured me the procedure wasn't necessary. I'd been so relieved, I hadn't questioned his decision. After three mammograms, though, it made sense to fully examine the lump. Might as well get it done soon and know the lump is harmless.

"Okay," I said. "We'll do a biopsy."

"Good. Let's set an appointment today."

I couldn't leave the office until I'd asked one burning question. "If we do the biopsy right away, will I be able to go to San Diego with my husband in two weeks? He's attending a business conference there, and I've been granted a leave from work to go with him."

Bob traveled often for business, but I was never free to go with him. This trip had seemed so exciting, I'd arranged time off.

"The trip may seem frivolous, but I've never been to San Diego. Everyone tells me how beautiful it is. There are special events planned for us, including a day at Sea World, and a moonlight harbor cruise. I've looked forward to this for weeks."

The surgeon grinned. "It sounds like fun. I'd like to go, too!"

"I hope I don't have to cancel. Bob and I are also planning to visit our daughter and son-in-law in Arizona. They're expecting their first baby."

Dr. Douglas' dark eyes were fastened on me. "Whether you travel will depend on the results," he said evenly. "If there's no cancer and no treatment needed, you should be recovered enough from the biopsy to go." *There's that terrible word again.*

"But if the report shows the lump is malignant, you shouldn't postpone treatment." Each word split the air like a rifle shot.

"This conversation's getting rather serious," I said, trying bravely to remain calm.

"Yes," the doctor agreed. "Staying well is serious, too."

I stopped at the nurse's desk on my way out. We scheduled the biopsy for Thursday—three days later.

The cold air outside felt refreshing. I inhaled a deep breath before opening the car door.

No big deal, I thought as I pulled away. I'll miss a day of work, learn I'm fine, and go on with my life.

* * * * * * * * * *

While I drove across town toward the high school, I reviewed the full calendar awaiting me. Thursday was the boys' basketball potluck, bridge club on Friday, the Sunday School party at our home Saturday evening, and Sunday, there was Sunday school and worship, then tennis that evening with Sandy and Page. My life was usually full, but this week was really crammed. I wouldn't have time to worry about the biopsy.

I wondered, though, what I would say to Bob. He often came home from the office in a dark, brooding mood. When I asked about his day, he'd say, "It was lousy. I don't want to talk about it." Some days, if I pushed him, he exploded like a whirling tornado. I'd sometimes react to his outbursts with silent, hurt feelings. Other times, I yelled back.

"No matter how bad my day is," I screamed one day, "yours is always worse!" I slammed a cupboard door for effect. "People you work with say you laugh and tell jokes, and make everyone feel good. They all come to you with their problems. But, when you come home, you're grouchy and moody! I don't think that's fair!"

Bob turned his back to me and disappeared to the bedroom

to change clothes.

When we dated during high school and college years, Bob was the class clown who performed Jerry Lewis comedy routines with his best friend, Larry. Bob even looked like Jerry, crew-cut and all. Today, at fifty, he was still witty, sensitive and compassionate. Our children had always sought his counsel. I never doubted that our love was deep and real. But I resented bearing the brunt of each day's turmoil.

"Why does everything at the office always look black to you?" I asked. "Surely something good happens once in awhile. You are good at what you do. Why can't you ever focus on the positive?"

"You don't understand," Bob said. "I'm always being second-guessed. You don't know what it's like to have people waiting for you to make a mistake."

I tried to grasp the enormity of his responsibilities and the toll they extracted from him, but I couldn't. I loved my job and never felt about it the way Bob did. For years I'd tried to counsel him and find solutions to his distress, only to be rebuffed. At last I realized Bob didn't wanted my solutions; he needed someone to listen and sympathize. If only I'd seen this sooner. It was too late now. We had given up discussing his work, and the stress had driven a wedge between us.

"It's just you and me now," I'd said after a bitter disagreement one day. "The children are gone, and we have to get along."

* * * * * * * * *

Trying to shrug off the upcoming biopsy, I worked the rest of the day, and met Bob at the kitchen door when he arrived home.

"Hi, Honey," I said, eager to see him, and hopeful, as always, he would be in a happy mood.

"Hi," he replied. He smiled half-heartedly, enough to create a ring of crow's feet around his dark brown eyes. His shoulders sagged; deep lines were set in his face. I snuggled against his tall, lean body and smoothed his gray hair with my hand. The smell of morning after-shave lingered on his face.

"How was your day?" he asked as he pulled off his wingtips and dropped them by the back door. "Anything new?" He draped his trench coat across a kitchen chair.

I took a deep breath. "Well, there is something. Dr. Spivey sent me to a surgeon today—a Dr. Douglas—to discuss the lump in my breast. He wants to do a biopsy this Thursday." My throat felt tight as the words spilled out. I reached for the refrigerator door. "I wasn't concerned, so I didn't mention it."

The distraught expression on Bob's face made me race on. "It'll be a simple procedure. I'll have a local anesthetic and be wide awake. There's nothing to worry about." I pulled open crisper drawer and retrieved vegetables for a tossed salad.

Bob continued to stare at me. "How long have you known about this?" he asked accusingly.

"Since last Wednesday."

"And you never mentioned it 'til now?"

"I didn't think it was important." I shrugged lightly. "I fully expected nothing would come of it."

He moved closer and slipped his arms around my waist. The look in his eyes was softening. My arms circled his neck. "I don't want anyone to hurt you," he said softly. We held each other and kissed.

"I love your kisses," I said.

"I love yours, too."

"Have I told you that before?" My fingers stroked his cheek.

"Only a thousand times," he said.

"Is that all?"

"Well, maybe two thousand."

We sat down beside the table. The salad didn't seem so important now. Bob reached for my hand and rubbed the back of it with his thumb. "I'll drive you to the hospital. I want to be with you."

"I'm glad. Dr. Douglas suggested you come." I got up and slid onto his lap and kissed his cheek. It felt good to be close to him. He was grinning now. I shook my finger at his nose. "Remember, this is a routine matter. You're not to worry until we get the results. Life is too short to worry, so promise you won't!"

He grinned again, reminding me of the Boy Scout he pretended to be in lighthearted moments.

"Okay," he said, "I won't worry."

But I knew he would.

As the evening passed, I found my confidence diminishing. Darkness was good for casting fear and worry on an otherwise positive mood. I lay in bed, staring wide-eyed at the ceiling.

This could be serious. Maybe the lump will be malignant. Maybe I'll die like Mother and Grandma. A shudder wriggled through me as images of illness and death raced through my mind.

My eyes teared as Bob's arms slid around my waist. I snuggled close to him. How good to know that, after nearly 30 years, his touch still comforted me.

I felt the beating of his heart. Constant and steady, like the rhythm of our love.

"I love you," I whispered.

"I love you, too."

Whatever the future might bring, I was certain the Lord would use my husband's loving embrace to transmit His love to me.

* * * * * * * * * *

It was Tuesday now. My boss, Mike, the Athletic Director at Moline High School, leaned against the door frame between our offices, sipping coffee while I stirred sugar into my decaf.

"I'm sure the biopsy is a routine procedure," I said lightly. "Everything has to be tested these days. There's nothing to worry about."

Mike shifted his weight from one leg to the other. "Yes, I suppose." He sighed and ran his hand through his short, reddish hair. His face bore the same distressed expression I'd witnessed yesterday from Bob.

Is everyone going to look at me this way now? Is it going

to be my obligation to assure everyone this is no problem? "Don't you worry about me," I said quickly. "I'll be back on the job Friday." Mike looked at me in a puzzled sort of way, but said nothing more before disappearing into his office. I thought how suited he was to the position of Athletic Director, having been an All-American athlete himself and a picture of health.

Seated at my desk, I pondered the upcoming biopsy. How I wished I'd requested more details about the procedure from Dr. Douglas. I was never good at asking questions of doctors. Now I realized I didn't know what to expect.

I began a list of questions for Mike's wife, Judie, a nurse at one of the area hospitals. She usually came by the office at the end of her shift.

When she arrived later, I asked her to step into the hall with me. I closed the office door and we stood outside it.

"The procedure sounds simple," I said in a hushed voice, "but I don't much about it." I shrugged lightly. "Shouldn't slow me down much, I guess."

Judie nodded and squeezed my hand. "I'm sure you'll be fine."

"Don't tell anyone," I urged. "I don't want people to worry for no reason." I motioned toward the office. "I told Mike, of course."

"We won't say anything," Judy replied. "We'll just pray that everything goes okay."

"Thanks," I said gratefully.

That evening I called our Sunday-school co-hosts, and they

agreed to have Saturday's party at the church instead of our home. "This is our secret," I stressed. "Tell everyone our house isn't large enough."

It seemed certain Bob and I would have to miss the basketball banquet Thursday night, mere hours after the biopsy. But I intended to play bridge in our couples club Friday. Later, we could decide about Sunday evening tennis. I loathed changing plans.

* * * * * * * * * *

The brown Oldsmobile sedan hummed quietly through the city streets. I was buckled into the center seat belt so I could sit close to Bob. Whenever I looked at him, he responded with a forced smile. It was early morning; traffic was light.

My thoughts were absorbed in memories of Grandma and Mother. Ugly memories, of illness and death. Leukemia had claimed my popular mother at age forty-eight. Grandma, the possessor of a Herculean spirit, despite her five-foot-two stature, died four years later. At age twenty-seven, with two young children and another on the way, I was left to face life without their guidance.

Bob said I was strong and determined like Grandma. "I has spoken!" he would say with a grin, an imitation of Lil Abner's mother, Mammy Yokum. Or he called me "Nora Ann" when I bristled like a banty hen who'd been challenged by the flock.

I sighed, thinking of the grief Grandma Nora Ann suffered from the deaths of her husband and two daughters. She could never mention the younger daughter's name without tears. After Mother's death, Grandma began her own battle with cancer. I remembered the recurring melanomas on her leg that reduced it to bone covered by a thin layer of skin. Finally, the cancer spread to her eye. I'd never forget that desolate night before surgery when Bob and I sat beside her hospital bed.

Maybe being like Grandma wasn't so great after all.

The car paused for a traffic light. I leaned my head against the seat. "Remember my 'going-away' dress when we were married?" I said suddenly.

"Sort of," Bob said, surprise in his voice. "What about it?"

"Did you know Grandma bought it for me? Mother was so opposed to us getting married she didn't pay for much, you remember, but Grandma rescued me and gave me money for that dress. There's a picture of me wearing it in one of our old albums, with my white high heels and wide-brimmed hat. I felt so special in that outfit!"

"You were special," Bob said. "And you still are."

"Thanks, Honey." I squeezed his hand. "Grandma also gave me the small white Bible I carried on our wedding day. I still have it in a drawer. She crocheted a beautiful handkerchief for me, too."

"I remember it."

"I carried it at Diana's wedding, and lost it somehow. I've always felt sad about that."

"Your grandmother was a feisty lady," Bob said.

"Remember how she was so possessive of that fancy cake

someone brought her when your mother died?"

"How could I forget? She nearly went to war with her neighbor because of it!" We laughed. "I wish she was here with us today."

"So do I."

"Grandma was a true believer," I said. " Her faith kept her going through all her heartaches. She always trusted God to help her."

"I'm trusting Him, too," Bob said. "Aren't you?"

"Of course I am," I said softly. "I know God is in control of my life and has been since I was seventeen and kneeling at the altar of the church where we were married." I paused to take a breath.

"What a wonderful day that was. Easter Sunday and the church was packed. Everyone dressed in Easter finery. The Holy Spirit must have pulled me from that back pew and pushed me all the way down the aisle."

Bob smiled and reached for my hand. Mine was cold, but his felt warm and comforting.

"It's hard to describe my feelings when I received Christ in my life. I only know that when I knelt in that church in front of all those people, I felt the presence of God within me. Nothing else has ever compared with that moment."

Bob smiled. "God is still with you today, as much as He was then."

"I know."

The Oldsmobile skimmed across the pavement. Bob

reached to turn on the radio, but impatient with the music, soon twisted the knob off again. I leaned back and peered into the morning sky. Except for the glare of occasional car lights and street lamps, everything was dark.

Heavy thoughts filled my head. Had I been foolish to be so nonchalant about the lump? With my family riddled with cancer, why hadn't I thought more about how cancer might affect me?

I'd been so healthy, it was easy to ignore cancer.

I glanced again at Bob. We smiled at each other. In the silence, I thought of our son and two daughters, far away. They'd be shocked to learn of today's biopsy.

Bob turned into the hospital lot and parked near the building. The dashboard clock registered 6:45. I reached for the door.

"No Long Faces!"

"Watch out for the spilled nails," a pretty, young nurse said in a loud voice as she ushered me through a maze of wall studs, eight-foot ladders and exposed ceiling beams. We stepped cautiously around piles of sawdust. The air was pungent with the aroma of newly-cut wood.

"Things are sure messed up, aren't they?" My voice was lost in the din of pounding hammers.

She shook her head to indicate she couldn't hear, then motioned in the direction of a makeshift dressing room. "You'll find a surgical gown and paper slippers in there," she said, her mouth close to my ear.

"Okay," I said with a nod.

The "room" consisted of wooden studs and unfinished sheets of wallboard. After undressing, I quickly scanned the area for the gown and slippers the nurse had promised, but none were visible. The nurse had disappeared, too.

I tossed my blouse loosely around my shoulders and peered into the hallway to find her. Fortunately, none of the workmen were in sight.

"I'm sorry," the nurse said when I located her in a nearby storage room. Her face was as pink as raspberry sherbet. "We're in the midst of remodeling and nothing is where it should be."

"It's okay. I'm sure being torn up like this makes everything difficult."

She nodded and reached into a cupboard for the slippers and gown. "I'm really sorry about the mix-up," she repeated.

"Don't worry. I think it's funny, and I needed a chuckle this morning."

Soon I was garbed in the elusive surgical attire and trailing behind the nurse toward the operating room. It was encouraging to see this room was intact and free of sawdust. A second nurse joined us there.

"You'll need to lie down on the table," the raspberry-cheeked nurse said. The surface of the table felt frigid and hard to my shoulders and hips.

"It's sure cold in here," I said. "My teeth are chattering." I could feel goose bumps on my arms. The cotton blanket spread over me provided minimal warmth.

"Most people complain this room is cool," Nurse Two said. Both women were busy and didn't seem inclined toward conversation.

While Raspberry Nurse fastened straps across my abdomen, Nurse Two secured my left arm to a board jutting away from the table. My chest was obscured from view by a cloth drape at my neck.

Dr. Douglas strode into the room. *Surgeons carry an aura about them*, I thought. *Especially ones as tall as this man.* Most of his face was covered by his mask and cap, but his eyes were animated and bright.

"Good morning," he said.

"Good morning."

"Is everyone ready?"

"I guess."

"That's good."

He stood beside me, a tray of instruments nearby. Despite the bright light above us, I continued to shiver. It seemed impossible to hold my icy right hand away from my leg, as I was directed to do.

I felt a needle prick; soon the left side of my chest was numb. I watched the doctor's face as he towered over me and heard him ask for instruments with mysterious names. The only sounds were his voice, the clatter of stainless steel and the snipping of scissors. I tried to identify the sensations of cutting and pulling against my chest.

"Do you feel any pain?" he asked suddenly.

"No pain, Doctor. But whatever you're doing really feels strange."

His mask quivered as though he was smiling behind it.

He worked in silence, then asked, "Do you have a family?"

"Yes, my husband, Bob."

"And children?"

"Two married daughters and a son—and our granddaughter. Diana and Kurt are in New York. Their daughter, Lauren, will soon be one year old. Tammy and Gary live in Arizona, and are expecting a baby in June. We're planning to visit them soon, if everything goes okay today."

"Yes, I remember we discussed that."

I wonder if I'll be able to go.

"Our son Terry is a student at the University of Illinois," I continued.

"Sounds like you have a nice family."

"We think so. We've enjoyed each other through the years." I was glad to be talking. It kept me from thinking about the snipping scissors.

"My husband and I grew up near the U. of I. and attended school in the little town of Villa Grove. I lived on a farm."

"I know that area," he said. "The land there is very rich, but very flat."

"Very flat," I agreed. "Much different from the Quad-cities."

I heard him ask for another instrument, then the room grew quiet again.

"Have there been incidences of cancer in your family?" Dr. Douglas asked abruptly.

"Yes, my mother and grandmother." A shiver slid down my spine.

"I'm sure you know cancer is genetically linked in families."

"For the most part, I've tried to avoid thinking about it."

"Breast cancer is the most common of cancers for women," he continued. "In recent years, mammograms have identified the disease much more quickly."

I wish he'd stop talking about cancer.

His words reminded me he'd said earlier that frozen tissue would be analyzed immediately after the biopsy, and we would soon know if the lump was malignant.

"Know any funny stories?" he asked suddenly.

When no one replied, I said, "I know one," eager to fill the void. "There was this patient who was about to have a biopsy and was forced to run around the hospital without any clothes. Can you imagine such a thing?"

Raspberry Nurse blushed again. I laughed, remembering my appearance in the hall, clad only in my blouse and underwear.

"That's not a nice way to treat a patient," Dr. Douglas said, a chuckle rumbling from his throat.

"It wasn't as bad as it sounds," I admitted, "but you asked for a funny story."

"We'll try to take better care of you in the future."

Will there be a future, I wondered as I struggled to keep from trembling. Raspberry Nurse squeezed my icy hand.

* * * * * * * * *

I followed Raspberry Nurse to the dressing area to discard the much-maligned gown and slippers. So far, this had been quite simple; I felt fine. Dressed again, we paraded to another small room. From the hallway I could see Bob. His eyes were closed, his arms folded across his chest. *He looks like he's praying.* At the sound of our footsteps, he looked up. The forced smile on his face did little to erase his worried look.

I hugged him. "I'm done."

"Great! You weren't gone long."

"Long enough. It was so cold in that room!"

The nurse turned to leave. "Dr. Douglas will join you later."

Bob and I sat down on vinyl chairs to await the surgeon. "Dr. Douglas talked about cancer all through the biopsy," I said. "I think he believes the lump is malignant."

Bob stroked my hand. "We'll see."

Within minutes, the doctor appeared. He was still wearing his surgical gown, but the mask and cap had been discarded. His easy smile was missing, too. In the cavity of my chest, my heart hammered a staccato beat. I wondered if it would burst through my ribs and explode into this bare, little room.

"The report shows the lump to be positive," Dr. Douglas said. I gasped for breath, but all I could feel was a raw rasping in my nostrils. How could this be true? Only minutes before we had laughed and joked in the operating room. Now his dark eyes searched mine.

"It is cancer," he said softly.

Oh God, please help me.

I stared helplessly at Bob. His face was etched with lines I'd never seen before. Was it fear I saw in his brown eyes? How could I have cancer when I'd been so healthy, so full of energy?

My body trembled as though I was stranded in a raging snowstorm. In my lap, Bob's warm hands gripped my icy ones. *Please, God!* I screamed in silence. *I want to live!*

No one spoke. What was there to say? All our thoughts were too terrible to voice aloud.

I turned away to blink back tears. In the uneasy quiet, memories from the past swirled through my head. Scenes of Mother, Grandma and Bob's mother. Images of suffering and death. They were so real, and this drama so surreal. Would their suffering be mine?

I strained to make sense of this madness. Is cancer the most terrifying word in the entire language? It seemed so now, cruel and deadly, daring to destroy my hopes and dreams. All the years of growing and learning, teaching and training were behind me now, and none was as powerful as this single moment that shadowed the air with doom.

"I didn't think it would turn out this way," I said at last.

"I know," Dr. Douglas replied, his voice soft and gentle. "No one ever does."

I studied Bob's face. He looked so weary and sad. If only I could spring from the vinyl chair to hug him and promise him I'd get well, if only I could make everything right. Instead, I sat in silence, still trembling.

Dr. Douglas spoke again, enunciating each word. "Let me tell you the good news. The lump is small, in an early stage. You are young and in excellent health overall. Much is in your favor to help you get well."

I leaned forward to absorb each word. Bob's hands held fast to mine.

"Breast cancer is the most treatable of all cancers," the surgeon continued. "Many women live full lives with only one breast." He patted my arm. "Go home now and rest. I'll see you tomorrow."

I watched him walk away, the unknown looming before me, unfathomable.

My life will never again be the same, I thought. From now on I'll be controlled by cancer and doctors and medicine and hospitals. A chill shook me.

I tried to focus on the doctor's parting words, the ones about living a full life with only one breast. They sounded hollow. I needed something more to hang on to.

Staring at the bare wooden floor, I prayed softly. "Dear Lord, please make me well. Destroy the cancer cells in my body. And fill me with your peace."

Bob pulled me into his arms. I leaned against him. "I love you, Honey," he whispered, "and I always will. Nothing will ever change that."

"I'll always love you, too, Darling." We stood clinging to each other.

At last, hand in hand, we trudged to the exit. Outside, the world appeared the same as before. Our car was parked where we'd left it earlier; others whizzed by us on the busy street. Above, patches of fluff drifted through the azure sky.

Nothing has changed, I thought, *except me*. In my head, a voice screamed, *Cancer, cancer, cancer.*

Bob began the drive home. I sat quietly beside him, re-living the hospital scene. How thankful I was to have not fainted or become hysterical. Given the circumstances, my calmness seemed amazing. Surely God was carrying me through this dreadful day.

"I'm hungry," I said suddenly, remembering I hadn't been allowed any breakfast.

"Me too," Bob responded. He pulled into a fast-food restaurant and ordered hamburgers and cokes. I gulped mine down.

When we arrived home, I urged him to go to his office. "Don't worry. I'll cross-stitch all afternoon." I motioned toward the half-completed quilt I'd begun for Tammy's baby. "I'll be fine. I'm not even sleepy."

"All right," Bob said at last. "If you insist." He hugged me and headed out the door.

Before I could gather my thoughts, Judie rang the doorbell. "You look fantastic!" she said, handing me a large plant nestled in a wicker basket. "Mike sends his love."

"Thanks," I said, surprised by the gift. I set the plant on the stereo, then hugged her. "I'm not fantastic, though. The report wasn't good."

She grabbed my hands. "Oh, Delores, I'm so sorry." Her eyes were filled with alarm.

"I'm sorry, too," I said quickly, "but I'll soon be fine again!"

She looked uncertain, but I hurried on. "I really feel sure

I'll be well. It was a shock to hear that report, but now I feel calm and confident I'll get well."

"I hope so," she said.

It made me feel better to proclaim good health, like all those times I'd tried to cheer Bob. Optimism came natural to me.

Judie declined my offer of coffee. I really didn't want any, either. We sat in the living room while I described the events of the morning.

"I can't believe you ran through the hall half-dressed!" she said with a laugh.

"What was I to do?" I asked, laughing with her. "I didn't want to put all my clothes back on!"

Was it amazing or foolhardy to laugh in the middle of a crisis?

When she stood to leave, I pulled her coat from the closet. "Thanks for coming. Bob and I will miss the basketball banquet tonight, but tell Mike I'll be in the office tomorrow."

"Okay, I will." We hugged goodbye.

After she left, I settled back on the couch and reached for the quilt. Pink and green carousel horses were taking shape, but I could visualize only the cancerous lump.

No wonder they call it " the Big C." It invades your mind as well as your body.

My optimism was waning. *Had a change occurred in the lump since the mammogram eight months earlier? Or were cancer cells there all along? Should a biopsy have been done sooner? Had I been a careless fool about this whole thing?*

One thing I knew above all else. In all my life, I had never needed God's love as much as now. I buried my head in my hands. *Jesus, I see you suffering on that awful cross. You loved me enough to give your life for me.*

A tremor swept through me, as it had on that Easter morning, thirty-two years earlier, when I'd met Christ at the altar of the church. "Thank you, Jesus, for your endless love," I whispered. "Help me to trust You now."

* * * * * * * * * *

Six years earlier, my friend, Sandy, a staff member at one of the area Schools of Nursing had given up her nineteen-year-old son, Brad, to cancer. I felt certain she could answer the questions that swirled through my head. I picked up the phone to call her.

Her voice was even, yet heavy with concern. "Surely you'll soon be well again. But I'm so sorry you have to go through this."

"Don't worry. I'll be fine," I assured her. I felt burdened to convince everyone.

"It's good you have a positive attitude."

"I guess, but the hardest part is having to tell other people."

"I know. But you can do it. You're strong." She paused a moment. "I hope you'll call Dr. Andrews, Brad's oncologist. He's an excellent doctor."

"I will," I promised, "but right now, I'm concentrating on this weekend. Bob and I may not be able to play tennis with you and Page on Sunday."

She sounded surprised I mention this. "Don't think about tennis," she urged. "Just take care of yourself."

"I'll do my best."

I hung up the phone and walked back to the living room. The quilt beckoned from the corner of the couch. I picked it up, then tossed it back.

Through the bay window, I saw dry winter leaves flutter across the front lawn. Was I a dry leaf, too, about to be blown away?

I bowed my head. "Lord, my life is in your hands. Please show me what to do."

* * * * * * * * *

"I've studied the lab reports," Dr. Spivey began when he phoned that evening. "The lump is in the second stage. First stage lumps are miniscule, while yours is slightly more advanced." I took a deep breath.

"I regret the lump is malignant," the internist continued, "but it is quite treatable, and your prognosis for recovery is very good. Don't lose sight of that. Dr. Douglas expects to see you tomorrow to discuss the various treatments available."

"Thank you for calling."

Bob walked into the bedroom and plopped next to me on our bed. He had listened to the conversation on an extension phone in the family room. His arms circled my waist. I leaned against him.

"Dr. Spivey sounds encouraging, don't you agree?" His voice was tender, and he seemed more relaxed than at the hospital.

"Yes. I'm sure I'll be okay."

He drew me closer. "So am I."

Our confident words sounded hollow, however, when I curled between the sheets that night. The air was heavy with one chilling thought. *I have cancer. I can't believe it's true.*

Memories of Mother, Grandma and Bob's mother crowded the long night. Friends like Donna, a gifted musician and teacher. Our neighbor, G. B., who laughed and teased. Jim, so kind and good. "The best boss ever," Bob had said. And Brad, his life ended so soon. Images of wasted bodies, blood transfusions and pain.

Would I be added to the list of cancer victims? Dr. Douglas and Dr. Spivey had each assured me I could be made well, but they couldn't promise anything.

Oh, God, please make me well.

Despite my fears, I clung to Dr. Douglas's words. "Breast cancer is the most treatable of all cancers, and many women are living full lives with only one breast."

I clung tightly to my husband, too.

* * * * * * * * *

"Wake up, sleepy head!"

I opened my eyes to see Bob. He was dressed in a suit and

tie, and smiling at me.

"I'm up!" I bounced to my feet and hurried through my shower before dressing in a red blouse, gray wool suit and high-heeled red pumps. I pinned a matching silk rose on my lapel. *Gotta look my best today.*

At school, it seemed as though I saw my office for the first time. "It's dingy," I muttered, "with its dreary concrete walls, battered cupboards and desk, and ugly green floor! Why do I love this place so much?"

Despite its dreadful appearance, I did, indeed, love this little room. The demands of the job had given me new life after the children moved away and left me with lonely, empty days. Today the office seemed to burst with confidence that the challenges and expectations it offered would play an integral part in my fight to be well.

One thing really was different. A new computerized typewriter perched proudly on the old metal stand beside my desk. Mike and I had ordered it earlier to replace my outdated model, but I hadn't expected delivery so soon.

"This is fantastic!" I cried as I flipped switches and experimented with keys whose symbols I didn't recognize. I felt as excited as a teenager with a new boyfriend.

What great timing. An unexpected rainbow in the midst of my storm. Surely this was a good sign.

I recognized Mike's handwriting on a note taped to the typewriter. "Welcome back," he had written.

Just then, he burst through the door. "Good morning," he

said. His face seemed drawn and troubled.

"Good morning." I watched him breeze past me and into his office.

A concrete block wall separated his desk from mine. I heard his chair squeak as he sat down, followed by the repeated grating of his desk drawer. Next came the roar of his pencil sharpener. *He's unusually active this morning*, I thought.

When the room became quiet, I called around the corner, "The new typewriter looks wonderful. I'll have no excuse for mistakes now."

Mike appeared in the doorway. "It's pretty fancy, isn't it?"

I nodded. "Had I known I'd be rewarded like this, I'd have been absent sooner."

He grinned, then looked distractedly toward me. He leaned briefly against the door frame, then retreated to his office. I stared after him.

How could I talk to him about cancer? What would he say?

I worked at my desk awhile, avoiding the dreaded conversation. At last I stood up and walked into his office. Pictures of Judie and their three children filled one corner of the desk. I sat on the lone empty chair in the room, opposite him.

Beams of light filtered through the window behind him and onto the desk. He looked up from a stack of papers, his face tense.

"I guess Judie told you the results of the biopsy," I said. I leaned forward to avoid the sun shining in my eyes.

Mike cleared his throat, then stretched back in his chair,

frowning as though he was in pain. "Yes, she did." He shook his head and brushed his hand through his hair. "I must be doing something wrong. You're the second secretary of mine to have this problem."

My body jerked in the chair. "Well," I said quickly, "I'm sure you had nothing to do with either of our malignancies. One out of every nine women has breast cancer, and we just happen to be two of them."

What made him say that? Does cancer come equipped with built-in guilt for everyone it touches? So far, I hadn't heaped guilt on myself; I was still too shocked by the diagnosis.

"I'll be out of the office this afternoon," I continued. "Bob and I have appointments with the doctors to discuss treatment."

"Sure, that's fine," Mike said absently. He swiveled his chair toward a file cabinet behind him, avoiding my look. "Whatever you need to do."

I rose to my feet. "Now, listen," I said firmly. My body trembled as I watched him turn toward me. The words spit from my mouth with a force that surprised me. "Let's get one thing straight. There'll be no long faces around this office. No one needs to worry. Everything's going to be fine."

Mike stared at me in silence.

I grinned suddenly and reached across his desk to touch his arm. "Okay, Boss Man?" I said with a laugh. "Do you understand? No long faces!"

His shoulders relaxed slightly. "Okay," he said, smiling. "No long faces."

"Good."

I hurried from his office to my desk, my high-heeled shoes clicking dramatically against the tile floor. I dropped onto my chair, my body trembling. The new typewriter awaited my touch, but I was lost in a jumble of confusion.

Mike is scared, and everyone else will be, too, when they find out. I suddenly realized what was ahead for me. Too much of my life was about to change. Too much was happening too fast. I didn't like change; I liked things the way they were.

But I knew the wheels of change had already begun to churn and I was helpless to stop them. Today I had glimpsed in Mike the depths of concern I would most certainly encounter in others. Today I saw clearly how much more would be required of me than merely overcoming cancer.

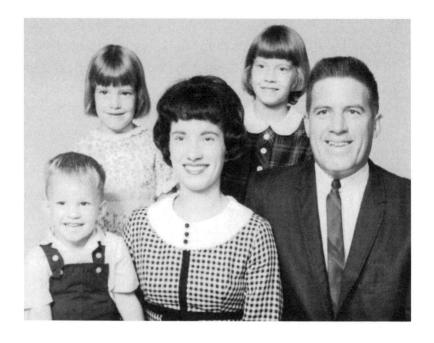

Bob and I and our three children. Left to right: Terry, Tammy, Delores, Diana and Bob. 1967.

I Could Cry

"If God is on our side, who can ever be against us?

Romans 8:31 LB

Bob's voice floated down the hallway like a soft breeze drifting through a narrow tunnel.

"Ready to go?" I heard him say.

"Almost," I called back as I leaned toward the dresser mirror and smoothed the collar of my blouse. *They'll never guess anything is wrong with me.*

I walked to the kitchen where Bob waited. "Don't I look healthy?"

"You sure do, Honey. You look great."

I winked at him. "You look pretty cute yourself." He was wearing the sweater I'd given him for his birthday, the one he chose every month for bridge club. "Maybe we should forget bridge and stay home to snuggle by the fire." Yesterday's biopsy and a busy day today were catching up with me. An ache pulsated down my spine.

"I'd like that, but if we don't go, they'll be short a couple. That wouldn't be fair."

"You're right."

I slid my arms into the coat Bob held for me. "Think we'll win tonight?"

He winked. "I'll do my best to win for you."

I wound my arm through his. "We've come a long way together, haven't we?"

"We sure have."

"Sometimes it's hard to remember the early years."

Bob's head shot up. It's not hard for me. I'll never forget those long nights at the chemical plant, and miserable days trying to stay awake in class!"

"That was a rough time for you, all right. Remember the day you drove thirty miles to college, fell asleep in the car waiting for class to start, and woke up in time to drive home?"

Bob shook his head. "That was terrible." We both laughed.

"It wasn't funny then. There were many hard days, weren't there? Maybe we should have listened to Mother."

"It would have been easier."

Mother had begged us to wait until Bob finished school to get married. I'd left college and lived at home again, and the mood in the old farmhouse was tense. Bob was midway through his junior year, but also "on break" to earn money to continue. My earnings as secretary to the County Superintendent of Schools were being saved for wedding expenses. In Mother's eyes, our plans to get married spelled doom for us.

"If you marry now," she argued, "Bob will never get his degree."

"He will, Mother. We know how important that is."

She wasn't convinced. "Just remember, when you get married, you're on your own."

"I know. We can do it."

As always, Dad was on my side. "Oh, Helen, they'll be fine. They love each other."

Four years and two babies later, Bob finally earned his Bachelor of Science degree. Having children so soon wasn't expected, and altered our plans for me to work while he attended classes, but by the grace of God we achieved our goal.

"Mother was very sick the day of your graduation," I said as Bob drove to our friends' home, " but she was proud to see you receive your diploma. She really did love you."

He nodded. "I know. How sad that she only lived two months after that."

"She was a year younger than I am now."

"That's so young."

"I never had a chance to resolve the differences between us."

We were stopped at an intersection. A motorcycle whizzed past.

"What a year that was. While Mother was so bad, Diana was hospitalized with a brain concussion and skull fracture after she fell down those basement stairs."

Bob shook his head. "It's a miracle we survived all that."

"It sure is. God must have kept us going."

"I'm sure He did."

We neared the home of our friends. I smiled at Bob. "Despite those hard times, I've never regretted marrying young. We grew up together and shaped our lives as one. And all those hardships made us strong."

Bob nodded. "We've had a good life."

I squeezed his hand. "Tonight will be fun, too."

* * * * * * * * * *

I always enjoyed bridge club with these friends. We had played together each month for years. Bob and I weren't the best players in the group, but we weren't the worst, either. It wasn't unusual for us to end up with high score. Good cards always seemed to run Bob's way.

Tonight, though, I was so tired I could barely tell an ace from a ten, let alone remember how many trumps had been played. The longer I sat, the more weary I became. It was a mistake to have come after the past tumultuous days. All my thoughts were on the afternoon conversation with Dr. Douglas.

"Your first choice is a modified radical mastectomy," he explained. Bob and I were seated across from him in the room where we had discussed the biopsy earlier in the week.

"As you may know," the surgeon said, "a mastectomy is the surgical removal of the breast and the tissue and muscle that surround it."

I took a deep breath. No, I did not know about mastectomies, and wasn't eager to learn. Especially when the breast and muscle in question were mine.

"Another option is a lumpectomy, where the lump and a

portion of the breast are removed." The doctor opened a book showing grim-faced women with scarred, misshapen breasts who looked like they'd posed nude for "Wanted" posters. I felt my neck twitch. Why would I want to look like that? I must have missed something in this conversation. "What's the value of removing part of the breast?" I asked.

Dr. Douglas smiled patiently. "Some women, mostly in the eastern states, prefer this technique. Locally, however, mastectomies are more common. You must decide which is the right choice for you."

None of these is the right choice. I like my breasts the way they are.

Dr. Douglas set the book aside. "The third option is radiation and medicine, without surgery. In some cases, this can be effective." Everything he said sounded so clinical and impersonal, as though we spoke of a frog in biology lab.

But this conversation was about me and my body, and what this surgeon might do to it. How would we decide? I was glad to see Bob taking notes on a yellow lined tablet.

"Each treatment has merit," Dr. Douglas concluded, "and all are beneficial." He avoided recommending any of the medical alternatives. "Go home and talk this over. You'll know what you should do."

It was late now, hearts and diamonds blurred before my eyes. I couldn't endure another minute of bridge club. Bob saw my signal to leave. "It's been a big week," I said to our friends. We hurried home.

* * * * * * * * * *

Beyond the bedroom window a Saturday morning haze hung in the air like filmy white gauze. Slowly I opened my eyes. What was this undefined sense of foreboding? The sensation reminded me of those days, years ago, when little Diana lay strapped to a hospital bed with a head injury. She had recovered fully, but the emotions from those frightening days loomed memorably in my mind.

I was awake now, aware of what was wrong. I have cancer. Today we must notify our family. I clutched the sheet and pulled it over my head.

Since I first learned of the cancer, I'd dreaded these calls. No one could be told face-to-face. Diana, Kurt and Lauren lived a day's drive away, near Rochester, New York. Tammy and Gary were twice as far, in Arizona. Terry was at the University of Illinois, 200 miles from us. My sister and brother-in-law, and my father and stepmother lived in our hometown of Villa Grove.

I pulled back the sheet and stared at the shapes of oak leaves embossed on the white plaster ceiling. How will we tell our loved ones I have cancer?

During breakfast I devised a plan. "We'll start with Deliece," I said. "Since she's a nurse, maybe she won't be so shocked." *Who do I think I'm kidding?*

How many sisters are identical twins? I wondered as I dialed her number.

The Cesarean section that saved our mother's life caused

Deliece to be born a mere minute before me. I always accused her of bossing me.

"Two little girls!" my father shouted as he leapt the hospital steps two at a time. "Joy Deliece and Jane Delores."

Most people called us "the twins," partly because "Deliece and Delores" was a mouthful, but mostly because they couldn't tell us apart. With duplicate clothing, matching shoes, socks, hair bows and barrettes, we looked identical at all times. We said "we," never "I," because we did everything together. Mother wished for a double wedding (which would have caused Bob and me to wait until Deliece finished nurse's training) but I preferred this day for Bob and me alone.

Deliece's personality was more steady and calm than mine. "Auntie is stoic," my children liked to say. People said our voices were alike, but when I heard mine recorded it sounded squeakier than hers.

Today her voice was heavy and drawn. "I'm so sorry," she said. "This is hard to accept."

"I know, but the doctors say my prognosis is good. I'm trying to focus on that. Most of all, I believe God is in control. It sounds crazy, but I'm not afraid."

"I'm glad."

We debated the various medical possibilities. "We're considering a mastectomy," I said. "That seems to be the best way to eliminate all the cancer cells."

"I feel that way, too," she replied. I smiled. Of course we would think alike on this.

"We have until Monday to make our decision."

"I'm sure you'll make the right choice."

"I hope so."

"If you have surgery," she said suddenly, "I want to be with you."

"That's great! Having you here would be the best medicine of all! Can you get off work?"

"I have some days coming. I'll work it out."

* * * * * * * * * *

It seemed appropriate to begin the calls to our children with our eldest. When referring to them, it was always in chronological order. I prayed for them that way, too. No matter what order I followed, I was always eager to talk to them.

For years I'd harbored dreams of life with my adult children, scenes of my daughters and me together, lunching and shopping, cooking and baking, sharing birthdays and holidays. I'd felt cheated of these times with my mother, and looked forward to sharing them with my children.

The dreams, however, had vanished with the moving vans that carried their second-hand furniture and treasured wedding gifts to new homes far away. They'd left so quickly—each daughter and husband within weeks of college graduation—I scarcely comprehended what had happened.

Terry had departed, too, off to the university in pursuit of his own hopes and dreams.

I had stomped through the tomb-like house. "If anyone else tells me what great places Arizona and New York are to visit, I'll scream!"

Bob reached for my hand. "I miss them too, but we still have each other. I haven't gone anywhere."

What irony! In the past I'd felt neglected by Bob's devotion to our children. Now he was all mine, and I longed for them.

I took a deep breath and dialed Diana's number. My hand held a death grip on the phone. This lifeline that kept us connected had now become an instrument of terror.

Diana's voice was soft and strained. It was difficult to hear her. Silence hung between our words like a rustling breeze on a starless night.

"The mastectomy seems the surest way to eliminate the cancer cells," she said at last.

"I think you're right, Honey. We'll probably decide to do that."

Bob had been quiet while I related the events of the past days. Now he spoke from his chosen spot by the downstairs phone. "Try not to worry, Skeez. Everything will be okay." She would surely smile at the sound of her pet name. I suddenly felt closer to her.

"We believe in the doctors' skills," Bob added, "and most of all, in God's power to heal."

The phone was silent again.

"I need to go now," Diana said. Her voice trailed off. "I love you."

"I love you, too," Bob and I said together.

The disconnected phone fell from my grasp. My body felt limp. I knew that in far off New York, Diana was crying. *This isn't right*, I thought. *I'm supposed to protect my daughter, not make her cry.* If only I could soar magically through space and hold her in my arms like I did when she was a child. I closed my eyes. *Oh God, please comfort Diana and calm her fears.* For long minutes, I sat in silence.

* * * * * * * * * *

When I went downstairs to find Bob, he was sitting on the family room couch. He looked as distressed as I felt. This is too hard," I said. "I need a hug to keep me going."

He flashed a look of mock complaint, but eased to his feet. His arms circled my shoulders.

"Do you feel big or little?" he asked playfully.

"Big."

"Tall or short?"

"Tall." We'd exchanged this banter a thousand times before. I leaned back to look into his eyes. "Won't you ever grow up?"

"Probably not. Will you?"

"I hope not."

Suddenly his expression was that of a little boy. "I don't want you to change."

"I won't," I said with a grin, "except maybe I'll get meaner."

Bob smiled. We stood together in silence.

"Is it time to call Tammy?" I finally said. I hoped he would say "No."

"I suppose."

"Oh, rats. You're no fun."

He grinned again. I plodded up the steps.

* * * * * * * * * *

Our younger daughter's voice was breathless with excitement. "We've been so busy getting ready for your visit," Tammy said. "We can't wait 'til you get here."

Oh, God, I can't stand this.

The sound of her voice ushered in memories of lonely days and nights. A ghost in my mind had heard the door open, but when I looked, no one was there. Only the silence of longing.

Bob had agreed to tell Tammy today's bad news. She gasped and, except for muffled crying, grew quiet.

"Oh, Mom," she finally said, "I'm so sorry."

My heart pounded as though I was caught in a cage. How much of this agony could I endure? These calls were all wrong. Our conversations should be joyous experiences, not moments of despair. I pleaded silently for God to supply the right words.

"Don't worry," I said brightly, "I'll be fine. One out of every nine women has breast cancer. I happen to be one of them." I paused to inhale. "Don't forget, God is in control."

"It's still bad news," Tammy said softly.

"I know. But it's not like in the past. There's so much new

treatment today. I'm sure I'll soon be well."

We fell silent. What else was there to say?

"Bye, Truffles," Bob said.

"Bye, Dad."

"I love you, Honey," I said.

"Love you, too, Mom and Dad. I'll pray for you."

I collapsed on the kitchen chair. Three down. Two to go.

* * * * * * * * * *

The call to Terry would surely be less stressful; men don't cry as easily as women. I'd cried enough for both of us after he left home. I'd even cried at the end of his final high school football game. Right this minute I could cry with longing for him, and I'd gladly launder his sweaty, grass-stained uniform again.

On second thought, that uniform was really disgusting after a sweaty practice in the mud.

I clearly recalled the years when the children were growing up. Terry had been involved in sports, and all three kids kept busy with church and school events, as well as part-time jobs. The calendar pages were so full I could barely find the numbers.

"It's like Grand Central Station here!" I sighed as teenagers swarmed through the house, inhaling chocolate chip or peanut butter cookies as quickly as I pulled them from the oven. In the laundry room around the corner, the washer and dryer roared continuously.

But I was happy with my life. Despite the frustrations and

demands made on me, my role as anchor in a swirling sea of activity brought me joy. My chosen occupation was that of caring for my family and supporting them in all they did. I was disturbed by those who urged women to seek new identities outside the home, claiming they needed careers in order to be fulfilled. Eventually I addressed the issue in a letter to the editor. "She's A Career Homemaker," the caption stated in bold letters in the *Moline Dispatch.*

"I do have a career," I wrote in part. "I am the local 'Coordinator of Domestic Affairs.' I have chosen this career over any other, and the pride and satisfaction I feel as wife and mother to four people who love, respect and cherish me is worth far more than any pay check or position."

During dinner the next evening, a handsome young man appeared at our front door. He was dressed in jeans and a jacket, and in his hand he held a bouquet of pink rosebuds trimmed with lace ribbon.

"For you," he said as he pushed the flowers toward me.

I shrugged in surprise. "I don't understand. It's not my birthday or our anniversary."

He smiled broadly. "I want to thank you for what you wrote in the paper. I plan to be married soon, and I hope my wife will have values like yours."

I felt the blood rush to my face. "Thank you," I stammered. "What a lovely thing for you to say." I glanced at Bob. He winked and squeezed my waist.

"Congratulations," I said to our new friend. "I hope you'll be very happy. You surely will be, if you treat your wife like this!" The man grinned and shook Bob's hand. We watched him walk to his car and drive away. In the years since, I'd never been able to remember his name.

My attitude toward parenting hadn't changed, but the circumstances of my life had changed considerably. When the children left home, I was lost without them. I had taught them to be independent, just as my mother taught me, but I hadn't known how much I would miss them, or how much my identity had rested with them.

After months of tears, I gained a new identity as secretary to the Athletic Director. Surely God had led me to the job, that I might have a new "career" and purpose. His plan had worked wondrously well.

I heard Bob's voice from the family room. "We need to call Terry," he said.

Okay," I yelled back. " Might as well get it over with." Having to tell our children about breast cancer was like pouring salt in a wound. I was glad to let Bob tell our son this news.

"Everything is going to be okay," I heard him say.

I couldn't refrain from joining the conversation. "Don't worry about me, Terry. I'm going to be fine."

"I'll pray for you, Mom," he replied. I heard a tremor in his voice.

"Thanks," I said. "I'm not frightened, but I need lots of prayer." After we talked awhile, we said goodbye.

I was surprised by each of the children's insistence that

they come home if I were to have surgery, which seemed likely. It would almost be worth the operation to have them with me. Almost. I shoved the phone aside. "No more calls," I said as I headed downstairs to Bob. "I'm too drained." He was slumped on the couch, staring across the room.

"Besides," I added, "I need to go shopping." His eyebrows shot up. "Well, I can't wear my old, faded nightgown in the hospital, can I?"

"Heavens, no!" he said with a grin.

* * * * * * * * *

The Sunday School group had become increasingly animated. I was glad to see them having fun with Bob's "crazy white elephant" game. He'd spent the afternoon planning this activity. It had been a good diversion from thoughts of cancer and the draining phone calls we made earlier. After my shopping stint, I helped tie strings around the paper bags Bob had stuffed with silly prizes.

The room exploded with laughter as each sack's contents were exposed. Bob was at his witty best, tossing out funny lines and teasing the older women.

I sat on a chair in the corner, watching the others have fun. Every inch of me ached. What was I thinking, anyway, to attempt so much in the two days since the biopsy? I did a quick review in my head: work at school; meet with Dr. Douglas and Dr. Andrews; play bridge; make stressful phone calls; shop;

prepare food for tonight; help host this party (sort of). I was paying for it now.

I looked up to see Kathy walking toward me. She would no doubt want to know why I wasn't participating. I'd have to make up some reason; I couldn't face her horrified look if I told the truth.

"Are you okay?" she asked gently.

"I'm fine." I forced a smile. "Just tired, that's all."

"You're so quiet. I thought maybe you didn't feel well."

"There's been a lot going on lately. I need a good night's sleep."

"Well, I hope you feel better tomorrow."

"I'm sure I will." I dragged myself from the chair. I couldn't sit here all night or everyone would wonder what was wrong with me.

Lord, I prayed silently, *help me get through the evening so I can go home and collapse.*

* * * * * * * * * *

There was little in my life more routine than Sunday morning worship. I'd grown up in a church-going family, and the weekly experience was as natural as saluting the flag in the Fourth of July parade. Some people thought going to church was boring or a duty to be endured, but I always left worship feeling renewed.

Kathy greeted Bob and me as we were about to enter the

sanctuary. "Are you feeling better today?" she asked. Her troubled expression and the anxious tone of her voice were evidence she was still concerned about me. I wondered why she so worried. Had the news somehow leaked out?

"I'm okay," I replied quickly. " I'm not so tired today."

"Good," she said. She gave me a hug.

I nudged Bob toward the sanctuary door and away from Kathy's imploring look. I couldn't tell her about the cancer. She would be too solicitous, too "poor Delores." I simply wanted to sit in quiet with my thoughts and sort through all that was happening to me.

Bob and I walked down the aisle to a pew near the front. His preference would have been to sit in the balcony, but he acquiesced to my choice of the front where I could see without tall people blocking my view. If our church was the indicator, jokes about parishioners fiercely claiming their weekly seats were based on fact. It was easy to spot different friends as we passed them seated in their chosen rows.

I slid close to Bob and reached for his hand. He clasped my fingers in his and rested them on his knee. I closed my eyes in order to concentrate on God's love. Slowly I felt the tension drain from me. In this lovely old building where we had long worshiped, I was safe. This was God's house, filled this morning with God's people. Good people, loving people, faithful friends. They would surely feel sad when they learned of the cancer.

While the choir processed in, I looked around the large, high-ceilinged sanctuary. Stately antebellum columns graced the chancel area and gave a sense of grandeur and majesty to the room. Colorful stained glass windows lined one exterior wall. More beauty was visible in the ceiling. I leaned back to gaze at light green glass panels trimmed with gold and ivory moldings. Hidden lights behind them gave the illusion of sunlight streaming through. In some panels I saw stained glass crosses. The effect was one of peace and calm.

I love this church, I thought, *it's neither too elaborate or too plain. It's just right for me.* Surely God was pleased with the look and feel of this building.

While the organist played the prelude, I closed my eyes and allowed my thoughts to drift, surprised to recall dark images of the past when our young family was transferred to Batavia, a suburb of Chicago.

"Just six months," Bob had promised. "Then we'll go somewhere else." It was November, and bitter winds turned the Fox River into a hockey rink, great for kids with sleds and skates, but I felt imprisoned by the century-old house we'd rented in this unfamiliar, frigid town. If only the phone would ring. If only I could return to the new home and loved ones we had left behind. If only there was some diversion from this boredom and cold.

Bob was as miserable as I. Each day in his first managerial position brought a new crisis. Our despair affected the whole family. "Whatever happened to love?" ten-year-old Tammy asked in a revealing poem. "Whatever happened to our family?" I felt so desolate I wondered how we would stand six months in this dreadful place.

"Lord, help us," I pleaded again and again. Tears streaked my face. It seemed God had forsaken us.

One night a familiar Bible verse penetrated my prayers. *There is nothing in all creation that can separate us from the love of God in Christ Jesus.* I sat up in bed, my body trembling. The words weren't new; I'd learned this passage years before. But on this dark night Paul's words seemed written just for me.

"Nothing can separate us from God's love," I repeated. Nothing! Not even this lonely, miserable existence. Shivers of joy ran through me. Now I shed tears of joy. "Thank you for reminding me, Lord," I prayed.

Soon other promises floated through the midnight hour. *I will never fail you or forsake you.* I lay bathed in joy and thanksgiving. Beside me, Bob was a picture of contented sleep. I knew God's spirit was with us.

I can face all conditions through Christ who strengthens me. With each promise of God's love ringing in my head, my hope for the future increased. We would survive this turbulent time. We would overcome.

And we had. Those six months were the most difficult Bob and I ever experienced, but we had survived them and—I could see now—were made stronger by the trials. In the intervening years I'd realized how much my faith was strengthened by those months of adversity. When we moved to Moline, I was once again filled with enthusiasm for what lay ahead. I smiled now, remembering the joys of these past years. All God promised had come true.

The organ music had stopped. Our minister greeted the congregation. I glanced at Bob. He smiled and squeezed my hand. I was grateful for his warm touch and this quiet hour to contemplate this new crisis.

A simple bronze cross on the altar drew my gaze. I stared toward it. The cross represented God's love through the resurrection of Christ.

In silence I asked, "Lord, will you truly never fail me or forsake me, as you promised in the past? Will you always be faithful? Will you give me strength to fight against cancer?" I believed He would!

During the time for silent prayer, I bowed my head. "Lord God, I praise you for your constant love. Help me follow you when I can't see ahead. Guide me, lead me, push me, pull me, drag me when I don't want to go. Don't let go of me."

After the sermon, the congregation stood for the final hymn. Across the aisle Kathy stood beside her husband, John. In an instant, I knew what I must do.

As soon as the choir processed out, I hurried to Kathy and ushered her to a nearby room. "I have breast cancer," I said.

She looked stricken. "I'm so sorry."

"I know. Don't worry. We'll decide tomorrow about treatment."

We hugged each other. "I'll pray for you," she said.

* * * * * * * * *

I sat alone near the phone in the kitchen, dreading this last call to my beloved father, Lowell Webster Woodall. Born on December 7—a day that would "live in infamy" —Dad was far too gentle in spirit to be connected with the horror of Pearl Harbor. It would be far worse for him to be connected again to the horror of cancer.

An image of him was clear in my mind—in overalls and denim shirt, leaning against the pasture fence, a hoe for cutting weeds in his work-worn hands. A breeze tickled the wisps of gray hair that circled his bald head; his blue eyes shone with a mixture of wonder and joy.

He gestured toward the long, straight rows of corn. He laughed to hide the emotion in his voice, but I wasn't fooled.

"I'm a lucky man," he said, his voice thick. "I'm free to breathe the fresh air, walk the black soil and watch the geese fly overhead. This is a wonderful life. I'm proud to be a farmer."

"And I'm proud to be your daughter." I hugged him, suppressing my own emotions toward the man who had given me a legacy of honesty, integrity and love.

Despite his devotion to farming, in his heart Dad was an author and teacher. He held a deep affection for great books and those who penned them, and his frequent use of the encyclopedias that filled the walnut bookcase in the farmhouse would have delighted any librarian.

When Deliece and I were young, he read aloud the poems of James Whitcomb Riley and a tantalizing story by Rudyard Kipling about a "curtious" young elephant on the banks of the "great, grey-green, greasy Limpopo River."

He admired great scholars and quoted them often. "A penny saved is a penny earned," he repeated to his daughters. "A place for everything, with everything in its place," was his standard for orderliness. That phrase, coupled with "Don't put off 'til tomorrow what you can do today," had no doubt contributed to my lifelong bent toward cleaning and "doing."

Dad was a student of life, too, especially farm life, and knew the leaf and bark of each tree he'd planted, and whether it had soft or hard wood. He was a fan of great achievers like Charles Lindberg, Jackie Robinson and Franklin D. Roosevelt (though he voted Republican all his life).

Thanks for a terrific childhood, Dad. It would be fun to turn back the calendar and be a child again, playing Rook, Old Maid and Checkers on a winter night.

My thoughts turned to my mother. She was a teacher, too, of the arts of cooking, entertaining and homemaking. Her dining table, set with china and crystal and decorated with fresh flowers from the garden, matched any Better Homes and Gardens cover. Her golden fried chicken rivaled the Colonel's. Her luscious desserts pleased many grateful guests. From her I learned to prepare tasty foods, polish the house and iron Bob's white shirts to perfection. Like her, I loved to cook and entertain.

Mother also taught about faith. "Lay up for yourselves treasures in heaven, for where your treasure is, there will your heart be also." (Matthew 6:20-21 RSV)

Her faith was severely tested during her two-year battle

with leukemia. No treatment was available back then. After Mother's death, Dad had married Dana. Throughout their twenty-five year marriage, we'd enjoyed a close relationship. My collection of 500 "love letters" from him bore testimony to that.

The sound of Bob's voice surprised me. So did the sight of dark shadows creeping against the kitchen wall. How long had I sat here, remembering? Much of me was in that old farmhouse; and much of it was in me.

Bob's hands rested lightly on my shoulders. "Is it time to call?" he asked. His voice was soft and gentle.

"I guess. We have to do this sometime."

My hand trembled as I dialed the familiar number. My heart pounded a staccato beat. Bob turned toward the family room. I heard Dad's voice on the line.

The hateful words were forced into being. Dad listened quietly. "Oh, boy," he said intermittently.

Were his eyes, like mine, brimming with tears? Was he reliving those difficult days before Mother's death? Was this too much for him to bear?

"Don't worry," I said quickly. "I'll be fine."

"I hope so, honey," he said softly. "I sure hope so."

"We'll call tomorrow night," Bob said quickly, "after our meeting with the doctors."

"Try not to worry," I repeated.

"I'll try," Dad said.

"Lots of love," I said huskily.

"Lots of love to you."

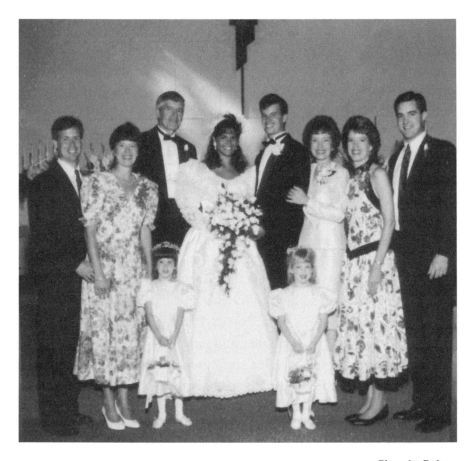

Photo by Robert

At Terry and Anne's wedding, August 24, 1991.

A Piece of Fluff

"In God I trust; I will not be afraid. What can man do to me?"

Psalm 56:11 NIV

Set back from the street in a residential neighborhood, Franciscan Medical Center could have easily passed for an addition to the high school across the corner. Bob and I drove past deserted tennis courts and turned into the hospital entrance. Through the car window, I stared into early morning darkness. It would be a miracle if the sun broke through the clouds today; March days in Illinois were notoriously dreary.

I stepped out of the car at the front door. *Here I am, the one out-of-nine woman who will soon become the latest statistic for the American Cancer Society.*

Why was I so lucky? I'd gladly give the honor to someone else. But I was the chosen one; number nine in line. No exchanging of numbers, please.

Bob held the hospital door open for me to enter the lobby. In his hand was my overnight bag with a few cosmetics and the new pajamas I'd purchased Saturday. I carried my purse, a novel I'd begun to read, and my Bible.

"Thank you, sir," I said as I walked past my husband.

"You're welcome, Ma'am." A casual observer might have surmised we were headed for a romantic rendezvous.

In the lobby, a statue of St Francis reached toward us with outstretched arms. His face held such compassion I wanted to touch his robe, like the woman in the Bible with Jesus. "Come, enter and be healed," he seemed to say.

How could that mean me? Though three doctors insisted this was true, it was incomprehensible that I was sick. If I chose, right now I could go outside and run circles on the hospital lawn. I'd be winded and tired, but not sick. Sick was someone in bed, feverish and weak. Sick wasn't an energetic woman like me.

I looked into St. Francis' eyes. *They say I'm sick. Please make me well.*

The elevator took us to the third floor. There, a partial repeat of last Thursday followed: draw blood, check blood pressure, fill out forms, use the restroom. Again, I was issued a thin, faded hospital gown, and told to sit on a gurney in the hall. The lightweight blanket around me only slightly warmed my shivering body. Bob squeezed my frozen hand. He had barely spoken all morning. I hadn't said much, either. It seemed we had talked enough about cancer.

A parade of hospital personnel passed by. Each one greeted us with a smile. The man who swept the gleaming tile floor whistled a familiar tune.

Dr. Douglas walked toward us, garbed in surgical attire. A paper mask dangled from his neck. I couldn't explain it, but some quality about the surgeon made me feel good, as though he were on the verge of doing or saying something mischievous. Even when he was serious, a suspicious smile appeared poised to spring from the corners of his mouth. Maybe it was his eyes; they often sparkled as though he'd just heard a joke. "Do you have any questions?" he asked Bob and me.

Bob's head was tipped to one side with his chin supported by his fist. His face was a study of concern. " How long will Delores be in surgery?" he asked.

Dr. Douglas glanced over his shoulder at the clock on the wall. "About an hour."

"That's not very long to change my appearance for the rest of my life," I said.

"I guess not."

We discussed the surgical procedure and anesthesia to be administered. I was given a consent form to sign in the unlikely event I required a transfusion of blood.

"Should I need blood," I offered quickly, "you could take it from my twin. She'll be here soon." I knew it wasn't possible for me to receive blood directly from her, but the possibility of receiving a stranger's blood was unsettling. Too many stories were printed about bad consequences from blood transfusions.

Dr. Douglas smiled. "I'll remember." He tapped my leg with his clipboard, then walked away.

A dark-haired nurse approached Bob and me.

"Ready to go?" she asked. Like everyone else today, she smiled graciously and acted as though we were her favorite persons in the world. I wondered if smiling and teasing were the first skills nursing students learned.

"I guess."

"Time to lie down." She eased me onto my back. Bob leaned down to kiss me. Above his smile, his eyes were dark and serious like his college graduation picture. I'd never liked that pose.

"I love you, Honey," he said.

"I love you, too." I smiled and hugged him hard. At last I let go of him.

The gurney rolled down the hall. I waved at Bob. He smiled and waved back. If only I could hang onto his warm, comforting hands. My whole body trembled as though I was trapped in a cold storage building. If I could go outside and run in circles I'd be warm. But the time for running had passed; there was no escaping now.

Why am I not crying? I wondered. At a time like this, shouldn't I cry? Tears came easily in the past when things went wrong. Shouldn't I be consumed with fear, my eyes red and watering? Maybe my tear ducts dried up or wore out, or maybe I'm in shock.

In OR (I was hospital smart now) a nurse strapped my arms and legs to the table. I had fully surrendered my freedom now. In reality, I realized, one has few freedoms in a hospital.

Another nurse tucked a heated blanket around me.

"Thank you," I exclaimed. "This feels wonderful!"

"Good," she said with a smile.

"Why is it so cold in here? Do medical people like working in cold rooms?" She shrugged in reply.

Maybe it's just me. Maybe having my breast cut off is the problem.

I'd been praying in silence all morning. For six days, actually, ever since the biopsy. I always thanked God for His love, followed by pleas for healing and strength. Prayer made me feel better. *Something would be decidedly wrong if it didn't*, I thought.

I recited scripture, too. "Trust in the Lord with all thy heart and lean not unto thine own understanding." What else could I do but trust? I certainly didn't understand why I was strapped to this frigid table, soon to give up part of my body. I hadn't a clue what the future held for me. I could only trust God to be with me.

Quiet sounds behind my head reminded me the anesthesiologist was preparing to put me to sleep.

The first hot tear slid from my eye and slowly made its way down my cheek. Then another, and another, silently streaking my make-up and falling like quiet raindrops onto my faded hospital gown. All the pent-up tears of the past six days, released at last into this cold, sterile room. I gulped air and swallowed wet salt.

I looked at the nurse and forced a weak smile. "I haven't cried yet," I said, "but I guess now's the time."

She dabbed my face with a tissue. "We don't mind a few tears."

The anesthesiologist attached an IV to my arm. "Count to ten slowly."

"One, two, three, four, five—" I no longer felt cold.

* * * * * * * * * *

Downstairs, Bob waited in a lounge with Dad and Dana, Deliece, two ministers and eight friends.

"We didn't want you to be alone," each one explained to my surprised husband. He shook his head in wonder.

So much for secrets.

* * * * * * * * * *

I tried to wake up, but whenever I opened my eyes they clamped shut again as though drawn by hidden magnets inside my head. At last I recognized Bob, Deliece, Dad and Dana hovering around my bed. Something about their expressions made me feel like a newborn kitten who had yet to mew. They all bore smiles of encouragement.

"Hi, Honey," Bob said. He gently stroked my hand.

"Hi, yourself." I peered through leaded eyelids toward the others. "Thanks for sticking by me."

"We almost had a party in the waiting room," Deliece said with a laugh. "You can't believe all the people who were there!"

"Dr. Douglas could hardly reach me when he came to report on you," Bob said. "The room was packed."

My eyes were slits again. "Tell me later."

"Okay. Go back to sleep." I wanted to sleep, but a seemingly endless brigade of nurses came to check my pulse and blood pressure and shine lights at my enlarged pupils. *Why can't they leave me alone?* Each time I awoke, nurse Deliece sprang into action. She seemed to know instinctively when I needed the bed adjusted to ease my pain, or the stainless steel pan held to my lips. "As soon as the anesthetic gets out of your system, you'll feel better," she promised.

"I hope so."

I was dimly aware of two plastic tubes dangling from my side with a collection bag at the bottom.

"They drain fluid from your incision to prevent swelling and discomfort," Deliece explained. "You'll heal faster with the tubes."

"Okay," I said as though I understood.

She pointed to the side of the bed. "The tubes are pinned to a sheet so the weight won't pull on your skin."

"Good." I dimly understood that I was held captive by these tubes attached to my side. "I guess I won't go far today."

"Not today," she agreed.

She held up a tiny spiral notebook. "To keep a record of your visitors and callers, and any flowers and gifts."

I watched with gratitude as she bustled about. "It's good to have you here."

She squeezed my hand. "I'm glad I could come."

When next I woke up, Mike peeked in the door. "Aren't you out of bed yet? The day's half gone." He looked at

81

Deliece and winked. She laughed. From the couch against the wall where Bob sat with Dad and Dana, I heard giggles. Mike edged toward the foot of the bed. "You'll be back to work tomorrow?" he asked expectantly.

"I don't think so." I tried to grin, but my lips seemed stuck together with putty.

He feigned seriousness. "The typewriter's in the car. Should I bring it in?"

The image forced a smile. "No, thanks. Not today."

Mike shook his head. "Well, if you won't come to the office and you won't type, I might as well leave. One of us has to work."

"Okay. It can be you." My eyes were closing again. He waved good-bye and disappeared down the hall.

* * * * * * * * * *

By midnight, despite the morphine drip attached to my hand, stabbing pain in my side and left arm forced me awake. If I attempted the slightest movement, waves of pain ripped through me. Deliece wasn't there to help me, nor was Bob or anyone else. I lay rigid, staring into the quiet night, praying for relief.

What, exactly, had this surgery involved? Everything had happened so fast, I felt ignorant of what had occurred. One thing I knew. The firm, nippled breast on my left side was gone and in its place was a straight red line clamped together by twenty-one staples imbedded in my skin and covered by clear, wide tape.

I lightly pressed my fingers against the tape. The only response was a sensation of pressure. Oh, God, will I always be like this? Will I ever feel life there again? I remembered Deliece and the other nurses commenting on the neatness of my incision. "Dr. Douglas did a great job," someone said. Neat or not, my breast was gone, and half of my chest was as flat as the book on my bedside table. *I'm not whole anymore; my body is deformed.*

Prior to surgery, when Bob and I discussed the matter, I made light of the situation. "It's only an enlarged gland," I said. "Removing my breast won't change who I am. I'll still be as impossible as ever."

He held me tenderly. "It won't matter at all," he said softly. "I'll always love you, whether you have two breasts or one."

But how could I be certain his feelings wouldn't change, now that my breast was gone? Would his assurances vanish when he saw the results of the surgeon's knife? Maybe our relationship would never again be the same. Maybe my body would be repulsive to him. I jerked with a sudden shudder. It was hard to think positive thoughts, lying alone in this hospital bed at night.

With my right hand, I reached to finger the cavity of my left underarm, surprised to discover a rope-like strand—probably a shortened tendon—stretched taut beneath the skin. The tendon felt strange, stripped bare of the muscle and tissue that had formerly surrounded it. How will all this cutting and shortening affect the use of my arm? Dr. Douglas had assured me I could still play tennis, but that seemed impossible now. Tears welled in my eyes.

"Lord," I whispered, "please don't let anything else change."

All the hospital was quiet at this midnight hour. Surely everyone was asleep but me. I wanted to sleep, but I couldn't. Dark thoughts tormented me. What would the morning bring? Would the pain go away? Would Bob still love me? Would I ever feel normal again?

Hundreds of people, maybe more, die of cancer each day. I thought again of Mother, Grandma Nora Ann and Bob's mother. Each of them endured great suffering, and yet they faced their illnesses with courage and grace. Mother had never wept in my presence, and only once alluded to her impending death. "I'm ready to go," she said on her final day of life.

But I wasn't ready to go! The only place I wanted to go was home with Bob and back to the world we shared. There was too much life in me, too much Nora Ann fight. No matter how the surgeon had carved on me, I was determined to go on living. His earlier words echoed through my head. "Breast cancer is the most treatable of all cancers, and many women are living full lives today with only one breast."

Dr. Douglas had cautioned me against comparing myself to others. "Each person's body make-up is different. No two patients are affected the same by cancer." He also said I would learn the results of lymph node tests before my hospital stay ended. Surely that report would be good.

* * * * * * * * *

"Ready for some exercise?" the chattery, laughing aide asked as she pushed a wheelchair into my room. "Today?" I asked incredulously. "So soon? When I'm in such pain?"

She no doubt had encountered this kind of response before. "Got the orders right here," she said, pulling a wrinkled paper from her pocket. "Your name's Delores, isn't it?" I nodded. "Well, then, let's get going!"

Why hadn't I known about this sooner? Had I not listened, or was this snippet of information conveniently overlooked? At any rate, my first session was about to begin.

All around the crowded therapy room stood odd-shaped machines and strange-looking apparatus. Each one was apparently designed to rebuild weakened muscles and fine tune dysfunctional joints. I sat quietly against the wall in my wheelchair where the aide had parked me. The trip from my room had been memorable as my courier laughed and joked with everyone we met. She made me laugh, too. If making others smile was her chief assignment, she deserved a raise in pay. She told me she was the mother of eight children, several of whom were adopted. I couldn't imagine that kind of responsibility or that degree of patience. You would need to laugh!

Across the room, I watched an older man attempt to steady himself with the assistance of two women and a chrome walker. His shoulders fell forward; his head hung to one side. With great effort, he inched forward.

Other men and women, clinging fiercely to walkers or

three-footed stainless steel canes, shuffled alone. In the center of the room, a young man lifted leg weights.

A small, young woman with dark hair walked toward me. "Hello," she said. "I'm Miss Myers."

"Hi," I replied.

She shook my hand and helped me from the chair. I noticed that she wore no make-up. In contrast to my wheelchair attendant, Miss Myers projected an air of seriousness.

She handed me a sheet of white paper. "Here are ten diagrams of exercises. Each one is designed to stretch and loosen your left arm."

The drills were illustrated by stick figure drawings. I looked them over. "They don't look too hard," I said hopefully.

Miss Myers demonstrated the first exercise. "Simply extend your left arm out in front." She made it look easy. "Do the best you can. Stop when you feel pulling on your incision."

I tried to lift my arm, but pain streaked through my shoulder. I reached for a chair to support myself. The room seemed devoid of oxygen. I took a deep breath.

How can a stick figure drawing cause such discomfort? I must be in worse shape than I thought.

"Why don't you try the next exercise?" Miss Myers suggested pleasantly.

"All right."

Figure number two held his arms high above his head. When I tried to copy him, the pain was intensified. I breathed deeper and glared at the therapist.

"Keep trying," she urged. It was obvious she wasn't going to coddle me.

I broke out in a sweat. Why am I being punished like this? Why couldn't I be allowed to rest and heal before beginning such strenuous movement? How could this somber woman expect me to perform these painful acts less than twenty-four hours since the mastectomy? What happened to my plan of being pampered in bed all day?

I studied the paper again. "Dumb drawings," I muttered. If they were real people, the day after surgery, they wouldn't be so smug. I was tempted to crush the page in my fist and toss it into the wastebasket. No one could force me to endure this pain. Was Dr. Douglas responsible for this misery? Behind his elfish smile there must be a sadistic mind.

Miss Myers watched from her desk. Obviously she was accountable for me, and if I quit, I'd be in trouble with her and Dr. Douglas. I had no choice but to continue.

At last, I reached the final drawing. It depicted the stick figure's hands locked behind his head and his elbows touching in front of his face. After several unsuccessful attempts, I turned from Miss Myers' watchful eye to blink back tears.

They're asking too much, Lord. Didn't they care that my arm dangled limp at my side? Had they forgotten about the tubes in my side and the incision in my barren chest? Beneath my pajamas, I was a perfect candidate for a circus freak show.

Miss Myers must have seen my frustration. She walked

toward me. "Take a break." She motioned toward a bench near the wall.

I sat down, the exercise page trembling in my hand. How could this sheet of paper be so formidable? These weren't geometric equations to be solved, or directions to climb Mt. Everest. These were just ink drawings shaped to look like people. I leaned heavily against the wall. My body ached; I felt weak. As I'd done so often in recent days, I remembered Grandma Nora Ann and all her hardships. She hadn't given up when the pain seemed too severe. She hadn't buckled under when the sorrow was too great. She had fought to the end.

Quit feeling sorry for yourself. This isn't the end of the world. You can do this.

I eased to my feet. Slowly, cautiously, painfully I attempted each exercise again. "Get strong, little body," I commanded. "You have a lot of living to do."

* * * * * * * * *

Bob was wearing my favorite red-striped tie and gray suit when he entered my room the next morning. A ripple of joy ran through me when I saw him.

"I thought I'd check on you before I go to work," he said. "I know it's early, but I wanted to see you."

"I wanted to see you, too. I'm glad you came." He walked to my side to kiss me, his lips sweet and tender against mine. "I miss you," I said softly. My arms circled his neck.

He leaned his head next to mine. "I miss you, too." For a long minute we held each other. At last he stepped back from the bed. "You look great, Honey! You even have make-up on already." He eyed me suspiciously. "Who were you expecting?"

"Just the doctor," I said with a laugh. "He always makes rounds early."

Bob grinned. "Well, I'm glad you're all prettied up, even if it wasn't for me."

"I'm glad, too. I even took my shower and fixed my hair. I wouldn't want you to see me all grungy."

He laughed. "It wouldn't matter. I'd love you, anyway."

"I hope so." I squeezed his hand and studied his fatigue-lined face. "You look tired. I know you've been run ragged these past few days."

"I'm fine. But life is pretty hectic. Lots of people have called to check on you." He kissed me again. "I'll be glad when you get home."

"I can't wait."

As I spoke, Dr. Douglas walked past the door. "Oh, no!" I cried.

"What's wrong?"

"Dr. Douglas is here, and I'm in trouble."

"What do you mean?"

"He told me to sit in a chair and walk in the hall, and here I am in bed." I glanced nervously toward the doorway. "I hope he didn't see me."

Bob laughed. "You'd better get up before he comes back."

"I know."

I pressed the button to lower the bed. With Bob's help, we maneuvered the tubes in my side and the bag attached to them so I could slide from bed and into my slippers. I was giggling, wondering if I had time to transfer to the chair without Dr. Douglas knowing I'd just landed there. Bob assisted me as I pulled on my robe, then helped me shuffle across the floor.

"We did it!" I said with a laugh. I leaned back in the chair and tried to act as though I'd been there all morning.

Just as I began to relax, Dr. Douglas strolled through the door. His ever-present clip board rested in one hand. On his nose, his glasses hung precariously. I noticed how freshly starched his lab coat appeared.

He shook Bob's hand before turning his attention to me. The familiar sparkle lit up his eyes. His lips and moustache wiggled quizically.

"You must think I'm pretty dumb," he said. He cast a knowing look toward Bob.

Laughter bubbled from within me. "I thought you didn't see me," I said with a shrug. "Honestly, I've been up and moved around a lot. Ask the nurse."

Bob winked toward the surgeon. "Don't believe a word of it. She was in bed when I arrived."

"This isn't fair!" I protested. "You two are ganging up on a helpless patient."

Dr. Douglas laughed with Bob and me. "All right, I believe

you. But from now on, I want you to stay out of bed."

"Yes, sir, I will." The conversation seemed to call for a salute, but I didn't.

* * * * * * * * * *

Funeral faces. They have me dead and buried already. I took a deep breath. *Lord*, I pleaded in silence, *help me make them feel better.*

The drawn, troubled expressions on the faces of a handsome, dark-haired young couple belonged to my son, Terry, and his girlfriend, Anne. They had just arrived from the university and were cautiously making their way toward my bed.

Their countenances were much different from what I'd come to expect in the past. Normally, Terry and I stood arm-in-arm, relaxed and laughing, and Anne and I eagerly greeted each other with a hug and kiss. Today they held their arms at their sides and tip-toed hesitantly across the room.

"Come here, you two, so I can hug you." I reached out my hand to pull them closer.

"Are you sure it's okay?" Terry asked hesitantly.

"Just be careful of the left side," I instructed. "Otherwise you can squeeze all you want."

Terry inched forward, with Anne close behind. "Okay, Mom, if you say so." He leaned down to kiss my cheek. Anne followed with a kiss of her own.

"See," I said brightly, "everything's fine."

Terry turned to see his grandparents and "Auntie" Deliece seated against the wall. "Hi, everyone," he said with enthusiasm. "Looks like the whole gang is here."

"We couldn't leave without seeing you," Deliece said with a grin. "You are my favorite nephew, you know." She gave him a hug.

"I'm your only nephew, if you don't count all those on Uncle Dick's side of the family," Terry said wryly. "Since they aren't here, that leaves just me!" Everyone laughed again.

Thank you, Lord, for breaking the tension.

Terry turned toward me. "We wanted to come sooner, but we had classes we couldn't miss. Now we're squared away. Our professors excused us the rest of the week."

"That's wonderful! I'm so glad you could come at all. I know how busy you are." They couldn't imagine how thrilled I was to see them, and relieved to have the momentary gloom dispelled.

Minutes later, the room exploded with excitement when Tammy and Bob walked through the door. Tammy's plane had landed a half-hour earlier, and they'd hurried to the hospital. She was radiant in a pink maternity sweater. Her face and hands were tanned Arizona brown.

I patted her bulging stomach. "You look wonderful, Honey!"

"Thanks, Mom. So do you." She leaned across the bed to hug me.

"I can't believe you're here. This is the best medicine of all!"

She smiled broadly. "I had to come to make sure you're okay." Tears suddenly brimmed her eyes. "I couldn't stay away." I swallowed hard. "Don't worry, Honey. I'll be fine. Having you here is sure to make me well."

I leaned contentedly against the pillow. Suddenly the nuisance plastic tubes dangling from my side didn't matter. Even the plastic tape plastered to my chest was forgotten. For now, nothing could detract from the happiness I felt. As though by magic, this room had been transformed into a refuge of hopeful delight.

A silly rhyme ran through my head:

Laughing faces; happy embraces.
Joy abounding; sadness drowning.
Thank you, Lord.

Two of our children were home again; the third would arrive tomorrow. All was right with the world.

* * * * * * * * * *

My first visitor the next day introduced herself as Jane Marshall. Streaks of gray highlights ran through her short brown hair. She wore a cotton blouse, dark skirt and low-heeled shoes, and appeared to be about my age. A canvas bag was draped over her arm. I was seated on a chair near the foot of my bed, reading a magazine, when she walked in the room.

"I'm a volunteer for Reach to Recovery, a support group for mastectomy patients," she said as she approached me.

"Thanks for coming." I motioned toward a nearby chair. A hospital social worker had told me earlier that Jane would come today. "Please sit down."

She eased onto the chair, keeping her head down as she reached for the contents of her bag. "It's been a year since my mastectomy, and this is my first visit as a Reach volunteer." She smiled weakly. "I'm a bit nervous."

I strained to hear her soft voice. "That's okay," I said with a smile. "We'll learn together."

From the bag, Jane produced an assortment of colorful brochures. "This leaflet describes various styles of breast prostheses," she explained. "There are many choices available."

She turned pages to show glossy photos of beautiful women in beautiful attire, made more beautiful—the advertising copy proclaimed—by the artificial breast beneath their clothing. I glanced absently at the pictures, surprised to feel goosebumps dotting my skin.

Jane turned to a second brochure. "This leaflet illustrates mastectomy lingerie and post-surgery swimsuits," she said. The pictures revealed full-cut, high-necked gowns trimmed with lace and swimsuits created with special pockets to hold a prosthesis. Their necklines with squared or cut in a high V design.

"I think you'll find the information helpful," Jane offered. She handed the papers to me.

I squirmed on my chair. "Probably so," I murmured. "When I get home, I'll study these."

When I get home, Jane, but not today. Not yet. *Please go*

away and leave me alone.

Jane, however, was in no hurry to leave. She might be uncomfortable with her assignment, but she was committed to completing it. With a deep sigh, she determinedly forged ahead.

Reaching again into her bag, she drew out a small rubber ball and a four-foot length of twine.

"It's important that you exercise your arm," she said as she walked toward the hallway door. "This is a simple maneuver you can do at home." I watched her drape the twine over the door, then grasp both ends in her hands and pull the string up and down across the door.

"This exercise will help you gain mobility in your arm. Want to try?" she asked hopefully.

"Okay," I replied carelessly, in an effort to be polite. At the door, I slid the string back and forth.

"If you do this several times each day," Jane said, "your arm will be stronger and less stiff."

"I'm sure it will help," I agreed.

Jane picked up the rubber ball and placed it in my hand. "Each time you squeeze this, you will build strength in your arm."

I squeezed the ball several times. Compared to the stick men, these exercises were simple.

We moved back to our chairs where Jane retrieved a small breast form from her bag. It was made of white cloth and filled with cotton batting. She placed it in the palm of my hand.

"I made this," she said. A hint of pride showed on her face.

"It's nice," I said weakly, wincing at the weightless, shapeless piece of nothingness.

"If you like," she continued, "you may wear this home from the hospital. Later you can decide which style of prosthesis you want to purchase."

Everything Jane said and did made me want to scream. I wasn't interested in her exercises or homemade breast form. Another day I'd think about a breast prosthesis and special clothing, but not today. I wasn't ready for this yet.

What was the rush, anyway? It would be weeks before the stitches in my chest and tubes in my side were removed, so dressing up and going out weren't imminent. As for going home, I'd simply hide my lopsidedness under my coat.

At last Jane rose to leave. "Thanks for the information," I said politely. Soon she was gone.

Alone again, I studied the flimsy piece of fluff in my hand. My flesh and blood breast was gone, and I knew there was no way in the world this pathetic wad of cotton could ever replace it.

* * * * * * * * *

I would soon be going home. Dr. Douglas had suggested I leave the previous day, but I didn't want to give up the magical bed and special attention from the nurses. I was amazed how attached we had become to each other in three quick days. They made me feel like I was their premier patient. Now, after three days of hospital food and a few more visitors than I had energy for, I was eager to leave. My bag was packed and Bob and I waited in my room for Dr. Douglas and Dr. Spivey to inform us of the lab report.

They strolled in together. After brief greetings, Dr. Spivey said, "Of the twelve lymph nodes examined, three contained cancer cells."

I felt the breath rush out of me. Oh, God, no. I looked at Bob. His face had gone white. In my head, the sickening words roared at a whirling, dizzying speed—like a spinning top—round and round and round in my brain. *More cancer, more cancer, more cancer.*

My legs threatened to buckle under me. I gripped Bob's hand and stared in silence at my doctors. How could they walk in here and, without preliminary discussion, tell me I have cancer in my lymph nodes, as though we were discussing what to eat for lunch? How could they do this?

I knew it took courage for them to admit that deadly cancer cells were lurking in my body, waiting to destroy me. They had, most assuredly, dreaded having to do this. Still, the news was enough to bring me to my knees. I swallowed hard.

"These ugly reports are becoming a bad habit," I said weakly.

"I know," Dr. Spivey answered, avoiding my look. "But three of twelve nodes is relatively low. Your cancer is quite treatable."

Bob shifted in his chair. I was amazed he could move. My body felt numb.

He cleared his throat. "Will Delores need chemotherapy?" he asked, echoing my thoughts.

"It's possible," Dr. Douglas replied. "Chemotherapy is often prescribed in situations like yours." He looked at Dr. Spivey, who responded with a nod of his head.

"I recommend you contact a specialist such as Dr. Andrews, whom you've already met," Dr. Douglas continued. "He'll advise you about treatment."

My mind was twirling faster. Cancer in the lymph nodes. Meet with the oncologist. Probable chemotherapy.

It was more than I could take. I suddenly felt outside my body, watching this scene from the corner of the room. Someone—it couldn't be me—was strapped onto the seat of a roller-coaster that twisted and turned, up and down, forward and back, helpless to stop. Would someone please pull the lever before the car careened off the track into a journey with no return?

Frightening images in my head drew me back to reality. I faced Dr. Douglas. "Will chemotherapy make me sick? Will my hair fall out?"

He looked squarely at me, his voice steady. "I suggest you call a patient of mine who recently completed 12 months of chemotherapy. Lynda has a strong, positive attitude, and can answer your questions better than I." He looked expectantly at Dr. Spivey.

"There's one more report," the internist said. I held my breath. "It's about the lump. The lab test shows it to be estrogen-positive. It's nothing to be concerned with now. You'll learn more about that later."

I hadn't the vaguest idea what he was talking about, and I lacked the courage to ask. Surely this fact wouldn't make a significant difference.

The doctors said goodbye and left. Bob and I stared sadly at each other. What bad news would we learn next? Would chemotherapy kill the cancer? Or would the cancer kill me?

I reached for my husband's arms. They were limp, as though drained of life. Still, his touch gave me hope. "Remember the words of Isaiah?" I asked. He nodded. "'They who wait for the Lord shall renew their strength; they shall mount up with wings like eagles; they shall run and not be weary; they shall walk and not faint.'"

Bob forced a gentle smile. "Those are beautiful words."

I looked deeply into his eyes. "God will give me strength to fly again. I know He will. And I know you'll take care of me."

"I'll do everything I can."

* * * * * * * * *

It was good to be home. Dad, Dana and Deliece had left everything in order before their departure the previous day. Our queen-sized bed felt almost as good as the fabulous one in the hospital.

I lay in our bedroom, resting and thinking. Down the hall, I heard voices and the quiet sounds of Tammy, Terry and Anne moving through the house. It was comforting to know they were there.

I couldn't relax, though; I was too puzzled by the lab report. It seemed each day brought a new crisis, a test of my faith in God. Would it always be this way? Would my life ever be calm again? Or would I have a life?

Suddenly, I remembered this was the day Bob and I should have flown to Arizona to be with Tammy and Gary in their new home. From there we were to go to California for days of planned activities and hours of fun in the sun. Tears rushed to my eyes. Other happy couples would stroll the beach and dine in fine restaurants, applaud the dolphin show or be lulled into bliss on a romantic harbor cruise. But we wouldn't be with them.

I eased to my side to stare silently into the dreary March sky. As I turned, my hand grazed the loose-fitting jogging jacket Deliece gave me in the hospital. It had a zippered front and matching pants, and with the drain tubes and collection bag tucked neatly inside, had been perfect for the trip home. I hadn't needed Jane Marshall's little breast form. No one was the wiser.

A gloomy eeriness pervaded the quiet bedroom. As I lay thinking, my hand slid under my jacket to the tape that protected twenty-one staples enmeshed in my skin. A fierce yearning caught hold of me. My arms clasped around my chest to stifle the shudder running through it; a salty tear crept down my cheek.

I shouldn't be here, God. I should be on the beach in San Diego instead of lying on this bed in Moline with twenty-one staples dotting the space where my breast used to be. Do you realize, Lord, that nothing is as it should be?

* * * * * * * * * *

Diana's voice awakened me. I could hear her in the living room, laughing and talking with her sister and brother and Anne. I eased from bed and shuffled down the hall, nearly tripping in my excitement.

"It's about time you woke up!" Diana cried. "I came all the way from New York to see you, and you're asleep!" I rushed to hug her.

"I'm so glad you're here. You look fantastic!" I hugged her again. "I hope you had a good flight."

"It was fine, or at least as fine as possible when you're wrestling a child who doesn't want to sit still."She looked at the floor where Lauren crawled among luggage and mounds of baby paraphernalia.

I knelt beside my granddaughter. Her eyes were wide at another unfamiliar face. Gently, I put my arms around her. "Hi, Lauren," I said softly. She looked to her mother for assurance.

"It's okay," Diana said. "This is Grandma."

"She'll get to know me soon. I'll let her play for awhile." I sat on a chair to watch her. She reminded me of Diana as a baby—thin and long-legged, constantly in motion. Her baby giggle was sweeter than symphonic music.

Miraculously, the distress I'd known earlier had vanished.

Who needed San Diego? Seeing and touching my daughter and granddaughter made thoughts of cancer, infected lymph nodes and an estrogen-positive lump (whatever that meant) disappear like after-school cookies. The coming week would be special, the house alive again with happy voices. We would forget every unpleasant thing, and bask in the delight of being together.

* * * * * * * * * *

When I called Lynda, Dr. Douglas' patient, I learned she was the mother of four young children.

"I'm getting back to a normal life," she said, her voice animated. "I feel great."

"I'm really glad to hear that!" I said.

"I was tired at first," she explained, "but my husband helped with the children, and overall, going through chemo wasn't all that bad."

"That's terrific! You're giving me lots of encouragement. I'm glad I called."

"So am I."

"Did you have any side effects?" I asked tentatively. "I'm worried about getting sick and losing my hair. I know that happens sometimes."

"Maybe I'm rare," Lynda replied, "but I didn't get sick, and I didn't lose much hair." She sounded upbeat and energetic. Anyone with four children would surely need lots of energy.

"That's great news."

"I saw a woman interviewed on television who said she vomited into a paper bag after each chemotherapy treatment," Lynda said. "One day her husband filled the bag with red roses." She laughed. "She couldn't throw up on the flowers, so that ended her being sick."

Mind over matter really works.

"Your optimistic attitude is just the boost I needed," I said. "I hope I've been helpful. Feel free to call again if you want to talk."

"I will. Thanks for the information."

Later, I repeated our conversation to Bob and our children. They were seated around the kitchen table. "Lynda sounded so good," I said. "She didn't get sick, and she didn't lose her hair. I hope I do as well."

"You will, Mom," Tammy said.

Suddenly I felt more confident. "You're right," I said, with a toss of my head. "Lynda's not going to be the only one who doesn't go bald or get sick."

I threw back my shoulders. "I can practice 'mind over matter,' too." My hands were planted on my hips.

"If she can be rare, I can be rare!"

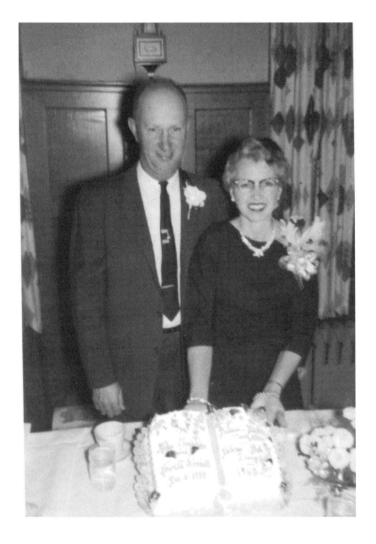

My parents, Lowell and Helen Woodall.

Chemotherapy and "Me"

"For my yoke is easy, and my burden is light."

Matthew 11:30 RSV

Our house looked like a florist's display room. No matter where I turned, bouquets of yellow astors, pink carnations, white daisies, green philodendron, fuchsia azaleas and bronze mums greeted me. An arrangement from my nephew and niece included a plush teddy bear.

The dining room and kitchen tables boasted centerpieces of fresh flowers. Other bouquets highlighted the family room. "If we light a fire in the fireplace, we'll wilt the daffodils on the mantle," I said to Bob.

He grinned. "I guess we won't have any fires for awhile."

I was amazed by the concern of others. "I didn't expect any of this," I said to Tammy and Diana. "I thought this would be a routine thing—in and out of the hospital, and on with my life." I shrugged in disbelief. "I tried to keep it a secret."

Instead of secrecy, the news had traveled far and wide. During my stay in the hospital, friends called and came. Since my return home, sumptuous dinners were delivered each evening to the house.

"It must be that awful 'C' word," I said to Bob one evening. He nodded absently, engrossed in the comic page of the newspaper. I was re-reading the cards and notes people had sent, enough to fill Bob's size 13 shoebox. I shook my head. "They're all so serious, hardly a funny one in this whole stack." Bob glanced quizically at me. "What's funny about cancer?" "Nothing. But I still need to laugh."

I thumbed through the mound of solemn, sympathetic greetings to find one from Sandy, the first of three I'd received from her. I held it up and began to laugh, aware of what was coming.

"Something about this card reminds me of you," I read aloud. The cover picture intimated a seductive woman in a bikini lurking inside. Instead, I opened it to see a wrinkled, toothless, cross-eyed old woman grinning contemptuously at me.

Each time I read the card I doubled over with laughter. "This is great!" I cried. Bob looked up quickly from his paper. "This card from Sandy means more to me than all the words of encouragement and promises of prayer I've received from everyone else."

"Really?" Bob said. "That's saying a lot."

"It's because this card reminds me I can still laugh—and that Sandy is laughing with me." I studied the card again. Beneath her signature, her husband, Page, had scrawled, "Play tough. It's do-able."

I lay the card aside and hunted through the box for another favorite. It was easy to spot the cover with its red roses artfully arranged in a handsome crystal vase. I closed my eyes to imagine the fragrance dripping from each delicate petal. Inside the card was a note.

"Why do I love you? I love you for the things you are and stand for while we are away, and for the things you are and do while we are with you." Other words of love followed. At the close, the author penned, "And now we will move through the door of love and happiness that leads directly to your smiling face."

From his home, hundreds of miles away, Dad had written of his love. Surely somewhere, Elizabeth Barrett Browning was smiling, or shedding a tear. Just as I was.

These cards, and all the others, represented so much devotion from loving, caring people. *It's unbelievable*, I thought. *I don't deserve all this.*

My thoughts sprang to a variety of support groups, such as "Reach to Recovery," available to persons who sought help. It was good to know they were there if I needed them.

For now, however, I had my own support group—an army of family and friends committed to aiding my recovery with food and gifts, cards and prayers, laughter and love. I wouldn't fight this battle alone.

* * * * * * * * *

Dr. Andrews appeared to be "fifty something," with a neatly trimmed beard and thick, unruly gray hair. He moved quickly, with a sense of urgency, the jacket of his suit flapping as he went. He motioned for Bob and me to sit across from his desk.

"We want to begin treatment soon," he said, his voice soft and steady. Behind his wire-rimmed glasses, his impressive blue eyes drifted between Bob and me. His manner suggested gentleness and compassion.

"We must wait, however, until the incision heals, usually about two weeks. Then we'll begin six months of chemotherapy." His words hung in the air like storm clouds on a winter morning.

I looked at Bob. His no-nonsense dark eyes stared at the oncologist; his mouth and chin had settled into a frown.

What was my expression? Dismay? Disbelief? Disappointment? I sat rigid on the chair, wondering what troubling information I would learn next.

Dr. Andrews leaned back easily in his leather chair. "Your chemotherapy will be administered in a four week cycle—a combination of injections and pills. You'll undergo two weeks of treatment, then skip two weeks." He reached across the desk to offer me an assortment of pamphlets. " Many of your questions will be answered in these brochures."

I looked curiously at the stack, then cautiously chose one entitled *Chemotherapy and You.*

My body stiffened as I thumbed through the booklet. Chemotherapy and Who? Was I really here, listening to a cancer doctor describe chemotherapy to me? This wasn't the way I had my life planned. My hands clenched involuntarily in my lap, the way they did more and more often these days.

"Take these home to read at your leisure," Dr. Andrews said. "Call me if you have further questions." He dismissed us with a handshake.

Later, Diana, Tammy, Bob and I (Terry and Anne were back at school) circled the kitchen table to study the brochures. In past years, I thought wryly, I'd spent much of my life in this room, cooking and baking, while the family stayed conveniently out of sight until dinner was served. Now we were gathered in the kitchen, and it wasn't even mealtime.

"Some of this stuff is gruesome," I said as I scanned *Chemotherapy and You.* "It says here that chemo can cause mouth sores, vomiting, loss of appetite and hair, and may produce darkened skin and fingernails."

"Maybe none of that will happen to you," Tammy said eagerly. "We'll all be praying for you."

"I hope you're right. I don't want to lose my hair."

The next paragraph offered less frightening information. "Drink at least eight glasses of liquid daily." I looked up brightly. "That'll be easy. I always drink lots of water." Tammy and Diana looked up from their brochures and nodded in silent reply.

I turned back to the booklet to read further. "Hmmm. This is interesting. I'm to be careful about scraping or cutting my skin, because, it says, 'anticancer drugs affect the bone marrow, decreasing its ability to produce blood cells. If the number of white cells in your blood is reduced, there is a higher risk of your getting an infection.'" I paused to read more. "I also need to wash my hands often, and avoid crowds and people who have contagious illnesses."

"Does that mean you have to stay home all the time to keep away from germs?" Bob said with a grin.

"No way! I'm going to keep doing everything I can." Tammy laughed. "I'm sure you will!"

The book listed other cautions regarding trimming nail cuticles and squeezing pimples. It stressed the importance of a warm shower each day, and admonished me to lightly pat my skin rather than rubbing it dry. Other pages detailed concerns of the mouth, skin and rectal area.

Which side effects will I experience? It would be horrible to lose my hair or be sick all the time. Across the table, Diana and Tammy were absorbed in other pamphlets. What were they thinking about all this?

I spoke again. "According to Dr. Andrews, patients in the past received chemotherapy for a year. I'm thankful they reduced the time to six months."

Tammy looked up from her reading. "Me, too, Mom. That will be long enough."

I turned again to *Chemotherapy and You.* "'Avoid aspirin, alcoholic beverages and direct sunlight while undergoing treatment,'" I read aloud.

Diana spoke suddenly, her face a broad grin. "I'll bet you're really worried about not being able to drink alcohol." She knew I never drank anything intoxicating.

"Oh, sure," I replied. " That'll be a big sacrifice!" We all laughed, a hollow sound designed to erase thoughts of chemotherapy and illness and future uncertainties. I passionately wanted to believe my chemotherapy experience wouldn't be extreme, but everything we'd just read described difficulties. Moreover, accounts of those I knew who had taken chemo were brutal. How could I expect to be spared a severe experience for the next six months?

I closed the book and set it aside. Considering the uncertainties of the days ahead, it would be a privilege to busy myself by cooking dinner tonight.

* * * * * * * * * *

It was midnight, but I couldn't sleep. Too many questions raced through the recesses of my mind. Though my breast was gone and loathsome tubes trailed from my side, I struggled to accept that my body was a seedbed for disease. I'd always thought God wanted the best for me, not acute illness. A verse from Psalms bore this out: "Seek your happiness in the Lord, and He will give you your heart's desire." (Psalm 37:4)

And what about that verse from Jeremiah? "'For I know the plans I have for you,' declares the Lord, 'plans to prosper you and not to harm you, plans to give you hope and a future.'" It didn't seem feasible that I could go through chemotherapy without being harmed. How could cancer possibly cause me to prosper?

A quote from a favorite Sunday school teacher of the past pricked my thoughts. "God doesn't cause bad things to happen to people, but He allows them." There were others who agreed, asserting that during bad times we seek God more. The concept made sense; I'd seen how God had used prior difficult days to soften and refine me, drawing my eyes and my heart to Him.

Other Bible verses seemed to reinforce this idea. "Come to me, all who are weary and heavy laden, and I will give you rest." (Matthew ll) Or, "I will lift up my eyes to the mountains; from whence shall my help come. My help comes from the Lord." (Psalm 121: 1-2)

Still, it was hard to believe God would inflict cancer on me just so I'd feel more need for Him. Couldn't He have found a less radical way to teach me? I never thought I'd gone so far from Him that He need employ drastic action to gain my attention.

At my next appointment with Dr. Douglas, I sought answers to my questions of "why?"

"All my life," I said, "I've taken good care of my body. I've exercised, kept my weight down, avoided alcohol and drugs. I've never smoked, and I've eaten enough fruit and fiber for a dozen people." I was seated on his examining table, garbed as usual in a paper sheet. I shrugged hopefully. "TV commercials say fiber prevents cancer."

Dr. Douglas smiled in his disarming way. "Those commercials sell lots of cereal."

Days later, when I met with Dr. Andrews, I put the same questions to him. How often, I wondered, had he heard similar words? His answer today was straightforward and simple. "We don't know what causes cancer, but we do know how to treat it." I thanked him for his honesty.

At home, I turned in my Bible to the familiar story of Job. In the throes of my own adversity, a refresher course regarding God's dealings with this righteous man seemed in order.

I discovered as I read that God didn't seem fair to His servant Job. Despite Job's constant obedience to God, the devil challenged God to allow him to test Job's allegiance. God agreed, and over time, Job lost everyone and everything dear to him—his children and servants, his oxen, donkeys, camels and sheep. Finally, he lost his health. The Bible said Job was "skin and bones," his loathsome body "covered with boils."

To make matters worse, Job's wife tormented him with less-than-sympathetic questioning. "Why don't you curse God and die?" she asked contemptuously.

Job replied simply, "When God sends us something good, we welcome it. How can we complain when he sends us trouble?"

I was amazed by Job's response. No wonder Job was looked upon as the epitome of faithfulness. He had seen past his misery and grief and defended God!

Despite his allegiance, curse after curse tormented Job, until finally, he, too, sought reasons for his sorrows. Had God abandoned him? His friends implied this was so. They even suggested Job had brought these punishments upon himself! For thirty-seven chapters, Job and his peers speculated about his situation. What terrible things had he done to deserve this misery? Why must he suffer so much?

I could easily relate to the story of Job and all those

"why's?" I always wanted an answer for everything. Why did our daughters move far away? Why must Bob be stressed out all the time? Why was I the victim of cancer?

At last, the Lord spoke to Job out of a storm, with questions of His own. "Why do you question my wisdom?....Where were you on the day I created the world?...Have you ever in all your life commanded a day to dawn?...Have you walked on the floor of the ocean?...Have you any idea how big the world is? Answer me if you know."(Job 38 GNB)

In the final four chapters, God asked Job many more questions, each of them demonstrating His dominion and glory over the world. Finally, Job meekly replied "...you are all-powerful...you can do everything you want...I talked about things I did not understand, about marvels too great for me to know...I am ashamed of all I have said."

The story of Job gripped me as never before, as new truths became evident. For one thing, I needn't be ashamed of questioning; even faithful Job had done so. It was normal to want to know "why?" But it was equally important to remember that God is God, the creator of the universe, the Lord of my life. He didn't owe me an explanation.

So, I realized, there would be no absolute answer. "The rain falls on the just and the unjust," I read in Matthew (Chapter 5: 45). God hadn't singled me out to suffer the indignities of cancer and its treatment. Neither did I believe He was punishing me for my sins, as Job's friends had asserted. But the rain was falling on me now, and the most important thing to know was that my loving Heavenly Father—omniscient, omnipotent, omnipresent— would fight this disease with me.

In the end, the answer to my "why's" was clear. I had cancer because the chemistry of my body was such that cancer could easily strike. It was as simple as that.

And the solution? Keep trusting God.

* * * * * * * * * *

My fingers clawed at the carpet above my head like a salamander burrowing in the sand. I was flat on my back, breathing hard, a layer of sweat beading my face. For fifteen minutes I'd tried to make the back of my hand lie flat against the floor, but it had refused to do so. I was almost to the point of defeat, but trying hard not to give up.

How would I ever master this elusive exercise? Was I doomed to live with a hand that didn't bend properly?

Those impossible stick-figure drawings. I wanted to strangle every one of them.

"It's no use," I complained aloud. "I can't do it."

A wave of frustration coursed through me as I recalled how I'd exercised my hand and arm religiously each morning and night.

From the quiet, the echo of my father's voice whispered in my ear. *Can't never did anything.* How often he had spoken this phrase to his daughters, encouraging us to try harder and never give up. But I was trying hard. I hadn't given up. And where had it gotten me? A pocket of air remained between the back of my hand and the floor.

The challenge from my father hung in the air like a floating balloon. I couldn't quit now. I had to keep trying, for him as well as for me. I gritted my teeth and extended my hand once more above my head. Stretching harder than ever before, I held my breath and forced the impossible into being.

"I did it!" I cried. Again and again I stretched and pulled, the touch of carpet against my skin as satisfying as the feel of rich velvet.

I jumped to my feet and danced around in circles. "I did it! I did it! I did it! Oh, God, you are so good. Thank you for this small triumph today."

The taste of victory fresh in my mouth, the time seemed right to attempt another elusive exercise. With my feet apart, I locked my hands behind my head and eased my elbows toward each other in front of my face. For the first time since surgery, they came together and touched.

A shiver of joy exploded within me. "Yippee!" I shouted as I dashed down the hall to find Tammy and Diana and demonstrate my successes. They laughed at my enthusiasm. "Great job, Mom!" Diana cried.

Again and again I repeated the exercises, delighted at my ability to perform them. "Nothing can stop me now!" I said. "This is a red-letter day!"

* * * * * * * * *

The house was quiet once more. This time, however, I wasn't devastated by the departure of our children. Terry and Anne planned to come again soon, and Bob and I promised Diana we'd drive to New York in June. When Tammy's baby arrived soon after, I'd fly to Arizona. I could survive the few weeks until then.

I sat alone, reading a magazine article about a mastectomy patient. Everything in the story detailed the woman's misery since her surgery. She said she hated to look in the mirror, and hid in her closet to dress and undress. She felt ugly and worthless. At times, she wanted to die. In every picture, she looked miserable.

Anyone reading this article would be terrified of breast cancer, I thought. Why must the media always focus on negative stories? They should have interviewed me. I didn't feel ugly or worthless. If anything, surgery had enhanced my determination to live a full life and look my best. Only Bob would see my body, and he assured me the mastectomy had not altered his feelings for me.

I pondered the story, challenged to reply, much as I had years before when cries across the nation urged women to forsake the home in favor of the workplace.

Instead of a written treatise, I decided today I would respond with action that demonstrated my positive attitude.

Rising from the couch, I walked to the bedroom to study my wardrobe. My appearance had always been important to me; now it had become even more so. A range of colors hung from my closet rod, with a predominance of blue and red. They would be good, but I shook my head at clothes that were black, brown or gray. "Sorry, guys," I said as I shoved them to the back of the closet. "You're going on vacation."

I grabbed a bright pink blouse and hung it on the center of the rod. Beside it I placed my favorite suits and slacks, the ones that made me feel attractive. I would wear these each day, accented with sparkling jewelry and sweet-smelling cologne.

I smiled confidently, aware of the importance of this plan. Never again would I be careless in my appearance. From this day forward, I would dress for success—the success of victory over illness—and conquer cancer with a confident attitude, a cheerful smile and vibrant, happy clothes.

* * * * * * * * *

It was Easter Sunday. Bob and I entered the sanctuary together, greeted by the fragrance of white lilies arranged in the shape of a huge floral cross on the altar. I turned to look for Sandy and Page in the balcony behind us. She saw me and waved. All around us, people were smiling and talking, animated by the joy of the day. When the announcements began we would grow quiet, but for now, we weren't very reverent.

Colorful banners lined the sanctuary, each depicting symbols of new birth. On one, a brilliant butterfly unfurled its wings. I was reminded of my own new birth on that Easter morning thirty-two years before. That had surely been the most important day of my life.

I watched the organist's hands skim across the keys, his feet gliding from note to note. His soul seemed to pour forth joyous sound.

The congregation rose to sing "Christ the Lord is risen today!" Bob held the hymnal for us. Every line of the hymn was a joyous affirmation of faith.

"Lives again our glorious King...Where, o death, is now thy sting?" My spirit soared at the wonder of God's love and the miracle of Christ's resurrection.

After the hymn, we turned to greet those around us. Everywhere I looked I saw friends who had written to say they were praying for my recovery. *Thank you, Lord, for their support.*

I was exhilarated by the hour of worship, alive with hope. The benediction at the end brought tears to my eyes.

"Surely it is God who saves me.
I will trust in Him and not be afraid.
For the Lord is my stronghold and my sure defense,
and He will be my Savior."

The First Song of Isaiah, Frank Noble White

Yes, God, I prayed as I slipped from the pew, you are my savior, and my stronghold, and my sure defense. I am not afraid.

* * * * * * * * *

Dr. Douglas examined the plastic tubing protruding from the small opening in my left side. With each visit, I'd begged to be free of this straw-like device and the collection bag at the bottom.

"It's a nuisance," I complained. "It dangles in the way and I can't sleep on my side, and I'm tired of wearing jogging suits."

He turned toward a table behind him. "We'd better get rid of it, then."

"Really? You're going to take it out?"

He smiled that playful smile that was so much a part of him. "I always do what my patients ask."

Within seconds, the tube was pulled from my side and the opening covered with a tiny bandage.

"You made my day!" I cried, fighting the impulse to hug him.

"Let's get rid of these staples on your incision, too. You're going to begin chemo today, aren't you?"

"I'm supposed to, if you give me the OK."

Using a tool similar to my staple remover at school, he quickly removed the staples. I didn't feel a thing.

He tossed his gloves aside, then reached for my hand. "Good luck," he said. "Everything looks fine. I wish you the best."

My throat grew tight; tears stung my eyes. I was saying goodbye to the man who had helped save my life. I wanted to tell him how grateful I was, how much his friendly, teasing manner had aided me through the past difficult weeks. Instead, I said simply, "I'm thankful for a good surgeon to help me get well."

A smile crossed his face. "Stop in sometime and say 'Hi.'"

"Maybe I will. You'll be surprised. One day I'll just pop in to see if you're still cutting up."

He laughed with a roar. "Okay. See you then."

I hurried to the outer room where Bob waited. "I got the drain out!" I cried, my voice suddenly loud.

He grinned and held his right hand in the air. "That's great!" I slapped my hand against his. Other patients looked up in surprise as the sound rang through the room like an exploding firecracker. I glanced over my shoulder at the receptionist. She was smiling. Behind me, I heard Dr. Douglas laughing in the hall.

We walked to the car. I wrapped my arms around Bob's neck. "What a relief to be free of the drains," I said. "Now I can start to feel normal again." He flashed a big grin.

"And I can wear real clothes!"

* * * * * * * * *

A nurse stepped to the corner of the desk and looked around the waiting room expectantly. "Delores Hackett?" she called.

I folded the magazine I'd been reading and placed it on the table next to my chair. Bob squeezed my hand and kissed me lightly. As with most of my appointments, he'd insisted on driving me here today. All across town I'd pretended not to see him glance at me and shake his head.

I stood up. "Well, this is it."

He made a jaunty thumbs-up sign. "I'll be right here if you need me."

"Okay."

The nurse directed me around the corner to the lab. I sat stiffly on a chair with my right arm stretched across a technician's work table. As instructed, I pulled my sleeve above my elbow so she could bathe the inside of my elbow with alcohol. She was friendly, and no doubt efficient, but I sensed a no-nonsense attitude, despite her soft humming.

Next she tied a rubber strip around my bicep. "Make a fist," she commanded. I clenched both hands, the one on the table as well as the one in my lap. To avoid watching what I knew to be coming, I stared at humorous posters and signs taped to the cupboards on the wall.

Suddenly the point of a needle stung my arm. I flinched and released the air in my lungs. The technician loosened the tourniquet, allowing thick mahogany-colored liquid to enter a plastic syringe at the needle's end.

I took a deep, determined breath.

"Are you okay?" she asked gently.

"I'm fine. Just need to catch my breath."

Before I could, she pulled the needle from my arm, taped a cotton swab over the puncture, then grasped my hand and sliced the tip of my finger with a sharp blade.

"Oh," I cried, inhaling quickly. A shudder ran through me. I watched her squeeze drops of blood onto inch-long clear plastic rectangles, then spread them thin with matching strips.

"All done," she said matter-of-factly as she taped a bandage to my finger.

"I'm glad this is over!"

"You can go see Alice now." Her tone indicated I should do precisely that.

Alice, a pretty blonde in her thirties, met me in the corridor. "We'll begin by checking your weight," she said pleasantly. Her voice was soft and sweet, and she moved with a grace that captivated me. Her entire demeanor made me like her instantly. I didn't like being weighed, though, and rarely stepped on the scales at home. If my clothes felt tight, I knew I had to eat less.

I stepped out of my shoes and onto the scales. "I always take off my shoes when I'm weighed," I explained. Alice slid the weight across the metal bar. I watched with clenched teeth.

"A three-pound gain since surgery," I said, shaking my head. "That's a pound a week."

Alice recorded my weight on a chart fastened to her clipboard. When she spoke, her voice mesmerized me. "You probably don't want to hear this, but it's common for our ladies to gain weight as they undergo chemotherapy. Their metabolism is affected and they burn calories more slowly." She patted my hand and smiled magically. "Don't worry about it. You can take off the extra pounds later."

She was right; I didn't want to hear this.

She left me to wait in a small room for Dr. Andrews. He

greeted me with the same friendly manner as before, my hand clasped warmly in his. His broad smile separated his gray beard from his spectacled nose.

"Your incision has healed well," he said after examining my chest. He had rolled a stool opposite my chair and sat facing me. "It appears you're making an excellent recovery."

"That's good news," I said. "I really feel great, and I hope to go back to work tomorrow, if it's all right with you."

"That's fine." He smiled again, his blue eyes lit with satisfaction. "We'll get started on chemo today." He rose and walked toward the door. "I'll send Alice in."

She arrived quickly, her tray laden with medicine vials, syringes, needles, gloves, a tourniquet and packages of sterile gauze. She moved with measured grace, carefully describing each object and its purpose as she placed it on the table beside me. Her soft, soothing voice hypnotized me, the way I was sometimes entranced by other people chewing gum.

She lifted the syringes from the table. "You'll receive Methotrexate and Fluorouracil—commonly called 5FL—by injection here in the office." She pointed to a vial of pills. "This is Cytoxan, and you'll take these each day at home." I remembered a listing of cancer drugs in *Chemotherapy and You*, and made a mental note to look these up when I got home.

Alice moved with an air of confidence, preparing the syringes and needles for my use. "I guess you've treated many patients," I said abruptly.

A sudden smile lit her face. "Oh, yes. I've been with Dr.

Andrews eleven years and have become well-acquainted with the ladies who come here. Until recently, we treated most patients at least a year."

"I know. I'm thankful I'm not one of them."

"Yes, you're lucky." She looked up, a delightful sweetness pervading every movement. "Many of my ladies have made full recoveries, and I never see them again."

I grinned at her repeated reference to her "ladies."

She filled a paper cup with water and handed it to me with a tiny white pill. "To prevent nausea," she explained. "The first treatment is always preceded by this medication. You may feel sleepy later, but don't be alarmed. This is the only time you'll need to take this."

I quickly downed the pill.

She tied a plastic strip around my upper arm, much as the technician had done earlier. With deft movement, she rubbed and patted the back of my hand until one vein stood up beneath my skin.

"Looks good," she said with a sense of satisfaction. She swiped an alcohol swab across the vein. "Now a little stick." I clenched my teeth and watched her nudge a baby-sized needle through my skin. "Okay so far?"

I nodded. Immediately, I felt the medicine crawling up my vein—warm and tingly, like a fuzzy caterpillar. Up it crept, inch by lethal inch. I could easily be deceived by this soothing sensation and forget its poisonous content. Alice emptied first one syringe, then another, into my hand.

Lord, please don't let me be sick.

Minutes later, she removed the needle and covered the tiny hole with a small plastic bandage.

"That's it?" I asked incredulously. "I'm done?"

She laughed. "All done," he said in her angelic voice. She tossed the used supplies into a waste can.

I felt my body relax. It was amazing how different the process had been from the tragic scenes I'd envisioned. *Maybe the entire chemo experience will be a picnic*, I thought. *Maybe I'll breeze through it without sickness, hair loss, blue fingernails or mouth sores.*

"Dr. Andrews will be in soon to see how you are," Alice said. "I'll wait until he comes."

Within minutes, he arrived. "How do you feel?" he asked as he pulled his stool close to me.

"I feel great! I can't believe how simple this was."

He looked at Alice and smiled. "We're glad to hear that." She nodded her head, then picked up her tray and left.

"Is someone driving you home?" Dr. Andrews asked.

"My husband is in the lobby." I shrugged easily. "He insisted on coming."

"That's good."

"I know. He worries about me."

For a few minutes we chatted as though we were life-long friends. He was so polite, so unhurried, so reassuring. His blue eyes reflected a life of devotion to people with life-threatening illnesses. I wondered how he could spend all his days treating cancer patients. Surely the stress would be more than he could bear.

I considered the gentle doctor and his experienced nurse. How many patients did they treat each day, this soft-spoken, unassuming pair? How many frightened people did they minister to with serenity and compassion? I only knew that today they had ministered to me, endeavoring to save my life. Tears of gratitude stung my eyes. I reached for a tissue in my purse.

"I appreciate all you're doing for me," I said, my voice thick.

"I know," Dr. Andrews said softly. "We want you to be well." The room was quiet as he stood up to shake my hand. "See you next week."

"Next week."

"Call if you have any problems."

"I will."

Bob grinned as I hurried toward him in the lobby. "It was easy," I exclaimed. "I feel great!"

"That's wonderful!" He stood up to hold my coat.

I hugged him. "Thanks for being here. I couldn't do this without you."

I Will Overcome

"Thou art my God, and I will give thanks to thee."

Psalms 118:28 RSV

As I'd promised myself, I was determined to look my best on this first day back at work. It seemed as though I'd been absent for months, but in fact it had been a mere three weeks since surgery.

Since surgery. I used that expression a lot these days. The term was a simple, non-threatening phrase to anyone unaware that behind those words the sinister, unspoken word *cancer* lay hidden. Most people took great pains to avoid speaking *cancer* out loud. I didn't much like saying it myself, nor did I relish the word mastectomy, which implied loss, lack of wholeness, illness. A softer, less epithetic expression like surgery made everyone more comfortable.

My attitude as I dressed for school this morning was more than comfortable. In truth, I couldn't wait to get back to work. From my "dress for success" wardrobe, I selected my favorite pink and white dress, then draped a strand of sterling silver beads around my neck, recalling the day the necklace—a gift from Mike, Judie and the coaches—was delivered to the hospital.

"I can see you now," I'd teased the gift-bearing coach, "standing in the hall by the gym, tripping everyone as they passed and demanding their money."

"You got it," he said with a laugh. "No one was safe."

The generosity of my co-workers had surprised me, but it was gratifying to know they cared. The necklace looked perfect against my dress. I was even more eager now to see these friends and thank them.

The dingy, gray walls of my office seemed alive today, reaching out arms and fingers of purpose—even love—to welcome me back. Memories of my first days here sprang to mind. The challenge and excitement of the work, the interaction with coaches and teachers, the opportunity to play out my fantasy of television's "Private Secretary" had effectively restored my self-esteem after the departures of our children.

Today, I felt certain, this job would play an equally vital role in my recovery from cancer. There would be no time for moping, no energy to waste on morbid thoughts, no idle hours to speculate on my future. The job would expect me to give it my all, without allowances for illness, slacking off or giving up. The job belonged to me, and me to it, and together we would forge ahead. Yes, I thought as I thumbed through stacks of letters and bills, this job will be good medicine for me.

Mike welcomed me with a hug, then motioned toward the new typewriter. "I've been talking to this machine for days, but it just sits there." We both laughed.

"Well, I'll soon fix that." I pulled off the vinyl cover and ran my fingers over the keys, instantly aware how much this instrument would elevate the quality of my work. A rush of excitement bubbled within me. What a fabulous way to be welcomed back!

I glanced around the office. No other changes or surprises were apparent. It was comforting to know everything else was the same as I'd left it, that no one else had attempted this job, that everything in this room had held its breath until my return.

One thing, however, troubled me. Despite the enthusiastic smiles and warm welcomes from my co-workers, their eyes held expressions of pity and fear, much like the worried faces of Terry and Anne when they first visited me at the hospital. Everyone said I looked great, but, judging from their eyes—where truth is always evident—they probably expected me to die.

Even the District Superintendent expressed concern.

"I'm fine," I replied when he "happened" to come by my office. "I feel great."

"That's good news, Kiddo," he said as he patted my hand. I'd never been called "Kiddo" before.

I'm not sick, I wanted to shout. Treat me the same as always. Two out of three women survive breast cancer, and I intend to be one of them!

How could I help others believe? Must I carry a poster proclaiming my wellness or plaster the office with banners of promise and hope? Should I cover my dress with some of the colorful slogan buttons I'd received, like "Classy Lady" and "God never fails?"

Should I recite the myriad of positive thoughts from the

Bible and other inspirational books I'd read while recovering at home? Was I the only one in this building who actually believed in God's power to heal? Must I be the one to convince all these doubters?

I cringed at the sight of their sympathetic faces. "God is in control," I said over and over. "I'm not afraid."

Some were more encouraging. "We're praying for you," they said.

"Keep it up!" I replied.

* * * * * * * * * *

I locked my desk, pulled my coat from the closet and flipped off the overhead light. The clock on the wall registered 2:30, one and one-half hours before quitting time.

"I'm going home," I called around the corner to Mike. I couldn't face him in this moment of defeat. Dr. Andrews had warned me of the exhausting effects of chemotherapy, but I wasn't prepared for its reality. Now, my fourth day back on the job, I knew. Tears of fatigue and frustration filled my eyes.

"See you tomorrow," Mike called cheerily from his office as I hurried through the door.

In the hall I breathed a prayer of gratitude. *Thank you, Lord, that Mike didn't question me, make sympathetic remarks, or offer assistance.* I had to get away, without any words.

At home, my positive thoughts unraveled like yarn in a kitten's paws. I threw off my clothes and sprawled across the bed, an ache throbbing in my lower back.

How can I go on like this, I wondered? I'd had more strength delivering babies than I could muster now.

"Gotta get relief," I muttered. I forced myself to the cupboard for pain pills, then hauled the electric heating pad from the closet and slid it beneath my back. The warmth felt wonderfully soothing.

I didn't wake up until Bob came home an hour later. He sauntered into the bedroom, a paper bag in his hand. "How about a sandwich?" he said with a smile.

I sat up to hug him. "You're a life-saver. I'm sure not in the mood to cook." I shook my head wearily.

He sat beside me and stroked my hand. "You look pretty beat. Maybe this food will revive you."

"I hope so. I'm wiped out." I shrugged sadly. "I wonder if my years of cooking have come to an end?"

"I'm sure they haven't," he said quickly. "But don't worry about it. There are plenty of restaurants nearby."

I hugged him again. "Thanks for understanding."

The next morning I felt refreshed and confident of a better day. By afternoon, however, my body begged for relief. I kept an eye on the clock and plotted to leave when I'd completed one last project, but just when I thought I was free, a coach dashed in with a paper that required typing. Next, I learned a team bus was late—call the company and find out why! And the phone wouldn't stop ringing.

So I gutted it out until the office closed. As each exhausting day followed, I realized the pattern was set. I would struggle through each afternoon, dogged by weariness and pain in my back. When at last I could go home, rest was all that mattered. My former active life had ceased. I gratefully spent the evening on the couch.

* * * * * * * * * *

I was more energetic Saturday morning—and hungry for deviled eggs, one of my specialty dishes. I made extra eggs to take to my friend and neighbor, Judy, who awaited the result of her own breast biopsy.

A plate of eggs in hand, I walked to her home.

She met me at the door, her expression a combination of surprise and delight. "For me?" she asked. She was about my height, with lighter hair and eyes, and a cheerful friendliness that was infectious. When you were with her, you were sure to laugh. I always said she made the best coffee and cookies in town. I was hoping for some now.

I thrust the plate toward her. "You can eat these," I said with a grin. "I'm not contagious."

"Whew," she said with exaggerated relief. "I'm glad to hear that. I love deviled eggs."

She rewarded me with a cup of coffee and a sugar cookie. "I'm not afraid," I assured her as we discussed my progress against breast cancer. "God is in control. He will take care of me."

"That's a great attitude," she said. Her voice grew wistful. "I'm anxious to get the results of my biopsy. It's murder having to wait."

"I know. I've often wondered why my report was available so quickly. Most women have to wait a few days." Secretly, I'd suspected my results were so obvious there wasn't need for elaborate screening.

"I should hear soon," she said.

"Call me when you find out. I'm praying your report will be good."

Days later I learned that Judy's biopsy revealed suspicious-looking cells. Her voice was upbeat when I called her. "I ate the eggs," she teased. "You said you weren't contagious."

I chuckled. "I didn't think I was, but maybe I was wrong."

"I sure hope not. At any rate, I'm glad you're laughing about this."

"You gotta laugh," I said. "My doctors and nurses insist a positive attitude will enhance my recovery.

"That's good advice," she agreed.

Soon after, I wrote on this theme to my parents:

"I feel like my life is not just my own anymore. Everyone is concerned for me, so I must make a "statement" of my life and and what I believe. Some days it's a strain to keep telling everyone, 'I'm fine. I feel great. There's nothing wrong with me.' But it's also a wonderful opportunity to say, 'God is in control. I'm not afraid of the future.' So I look as good as I can every day, and wear bright buttons that read, 'Hang in There,' or 'Put on a Happy Face.' I'm determined to go on with my life as always."

After more tests and minor surgery, Judy was declared "cancer-free." I hoped my confident attitude had been an encouragement to her. I was certain it was aiding my own recovery.

* * * * * * * * * *

The tennis racquet felt good in my hand. I'd pulled it from the closet and was swinging it back and forth when Bob walked into the living room.

"Are you sure you're ready for this?" he asked, his eyebrow arched. "It's been less than four weeks since surgery, and only days since you began chemo. And you've been exhausted all week." His expression suggested I'd lost my mind.

"I know, but I'm not a bit tired today, and I really want to play. Besides, Dr. Douglas said it's okay." I swung the racquet again. "My arm isn't sore or tight. All those exercises really paid off!"

"Okay," he said with a sigh. "No sense arguing."

At the high school courts, I propped my water bottle near the net, then bounced eagerly onto the court. Bob sauntered to the opposite side.

I looked excitedly toward my husband. With his twelve-inch height advantage and the fact he'd played high school and college sports, it was obvious he could beat me blindfolded any day. Even so, I always approached our matches in the same way I confronted life—with full confidence I could win.

We began with routine shots. Before long, though, we were trading drop shots and lobs. I was bursting with joy to be back on the court. Bob drove me from corner to corner, alley to alley, baseline to net.

"This is great!" I yelled as I blasted the ball down the baseline with a two-fisted backhand. "I don't feel a bit tired!" He laughed, an infectious giggle that burst through the spring air and bounced off nearby trees. I was thrilled to hear him laughing, knowing how sad he'd looked all week when he found me sprawled across the bed or living room couch.

Sweat dripped from my face and neck. The fuzzy, yellow orb sailed back and forth—my side, his side, over and back again. *I will overcome!* it seemed to shout.

I glanced at my watch; we'd played for an hour. I waited in the backcourt to receive his serve. The amber sphere exploded from my racquet. I watched with satisfaction as it sailed deep into his corner. He ran futilely toward it, turning to flash a "thumbs up" sign as he went.

"Got you that time!" I shouted. In my chest, my heart pounded, *I will overcome!*

Bob served once more, quickly charging the net where he usually intercepted my return. Instead, I lobbed the ball over his head to land inches inside the baseline. "Great shot!" he cried. His face bore a look of glee.

"Yeah for me!" I shouted as I ran toward the net, my racquet high above my head. I waved it back and forth. "My banner of triumph!" I cried. We laughed joyously. "I will overcome!"

Bob opened his arms to embrace me. "I know you will." Suddenly I recalled Page's note after surgery. "It's doable," he'd written.

In this instant, exhilarated by this hour of tennis, I knew he was right. I had faced unfathomed challenges the past few weeks. My life had been turned upside down. In spite of everything, I was doing it.

Had I been standing at the summit of Mt. Everest, I couldn't have felt higher.

* * * * * * * * * *

We met Sandy and Page at the tennis club—a huge structure that housed three courts, an exercise area and snack bar—the next evening. Prior to joining a woman's league at the club years before, my tennis consisted of summer park programs and playing against Bob on neighborhood courts. It had been enormously gratifying to know I could compete satisfactorily against other women.

Bob and I took our places on the court across from Sandy and Page.

"You look great!" Sandy praised. "You haven't slowed down a bit!"

"Wait 'til tomorrow," I warned. "I'll be a zombie again."

All through the hour I felt energized and enthused. Knowing I had full use of my arm and upper body sent adrenaline rushing through me. My worst fears were proven wrong. No matter what had occurred in the cells that made up my body, I was still strong and vibrant, physically and mentally capable of playing tennis. Throughout the match I repeatedly praised God for this victory.

In the locker room later, I was surprised to discover Sandy in the far corner of the dressing room with rows of tall lockers between us. In the past, we'd always dressed near each other.

After my shower I sought her out. She was bent over, tying her shoes. "Would you like to see my scar?" I asked abruptly.

She looked up hesitantly. "Okay, if you want to show me."

"Since you're a nurse," I explained, "I thought you'd appreciate how well the incision has healed." I unbuttoned my blouse to reveal the scar.

Sandy glanced at the incision, then back at her feet. "You're right," she said, her head down, "it has healed very well."

"I think so."

She looked up and smiled weakly. "You're off to a good start."

"I hope so."

I returned to my locker, confused by her guarded response. Sandy was usually animated and exuberant. My actions today must had made her uncomfortable, perhaps embarrassed. Would she have reacted differently if the scar had been on my stomach? Probably. But stomach surgery didn't substantially change one's appearance.

I wanted to believe my incision was simply a scar, a closure binding together two pieces of flesh. In truth, however, the scar represented cancer, disfigurement and loss—difficult criteria to accept. Even Sandy, a nurse and close friend, would have preferred I not draw her into my cancer experience. I couldn't blame her; she'd endured enough cancer agony with her son, Brad. The harsh truth was that my mastectomy, or surgery, or cancer— whichever term I chose to use—had once again set me apart. My body was changed, and so was I. No longer could I deny this. I'd have to accept the changes I desperately yearned to avoid.

* * * * * * * * * *

Sandy's wasn't the only attitude to have changed; co-workers exhibited an "attitude adjustment" as well. It was almost comical to see doors held open as I approached, and to have my smile greeted with greater affection than before. My opinions suddenly garnered more consideration than in the past. When I asked for something, I usually got it. *Pamper this woman*, the actions of those around me suggested—she's engaged in a battle for her life.

I was uncomfortable with so much patronage, but a portion of me enjoyed all the fuss. Who doesn't enjoy being pampered? I might be a "Mammy Yokum" at times, but I was also a frills-and-lace female, clad in high-heeled shoes and gold-plated chains. It was fun to be waited on and made to feel more important. At the same time, I wanted to be liked and appreciated for myself and my abilities, not because cancer cells lurked within me. I tried not to take advantage of my favored position.

I was especially aware that my current status created new opportunities in regard to my faith. For years I'd prayed to be a witness to God's love, but—like many others—I was reluctant to verbalize my feelings for fear of misunderstanding or ridicule or alienation from others.

Now, people were watching me like fireworks on the Fourth of July. How was I reacting to this crisis? Was I caving in? Was fear overwhelming me?

To those who wondered whether God really would make a difference in my cancer experience, I said, "His presence enables me to go on with hope. His power gives me strength despite the physical weariness and uncertainties of this disease."

Over and over I said, "God is in control. I'm not afraid." And in my prayers, I asked God to use my illness to draw others to Him.

* * * * * * * * *

Even without my blazer and shoes—which I had quickly discarded—the Medical Arts scale reflected a two-pound gain since my last appointment, which meant an increase since surgery of five pounds.

I frowned at Alice. "If I add two pounds each time I come, by the end of six months I'll be too fat to wear any of my clothes!" Already, too-tight waistbands struggled to meet and zippers refused to close. Control-top pantyhose had become a form of torture.

Alice slid the weights back to prevent my further glares. "Remember," she said sweetly, "most patients gain weight during treatment. Some of the ladies have gone to dieticians and arranged special diets, but still gained extra pounds. Try not to worry too much about it."

That's easy for you to say. I surveyed her slim body, which appeared to be a size six. At the rate I was going, I would soon be a size 20. How could I satisfy my energy-starved body without over-eating?

"Try raw carrot sticks for between-meal snacks," Dr. Andrews suggested when I asked him, "and leave the dressings off your green salads."

The carrots were tasty and nutritional, with enough sugar to provide an energy boost. Orange juice, soda crackers or a graham cracker helped satisfy my mid-morning cravings, and the mixture of nuts, raisins and seeds stashed in my desk drawer served as great "pick-me-up's" anytime. For lunch, I ate low-fat cottage cheese or water-packed tuna (straight from the can) with fresh fruit and skim milk. Junk food and desserts were no-no's.

Despite my efforts, the pounds crept upward.

"I hate this extra weight!" I complained to Sandy at tennis. "No matter how hard I try, I can't keep it under control."

She seemed baffled by my concern. "I think you look great. I can't see any difference."

I shrugged in dismay. "Everything's too tight around my waist. It's so frustrating!"

One Sunday evening, after listening to my complaints for weeks, she offered me a package wrapped in newsprint and tied with string. I looked at her quizzically. This wasn't typical of my well-mannered friend. Her expression reminded me of the Siamese cats in *Lady and the Tramp* as they pounced on the dog.

Inside the paper I discovered an enormous, multi-colored cotton dress. "You shouldn't have!" I exclaimed as I spread the dress in front of me. Red and yellow flowers stared up at me. The garment was large enough to cover Sandy and me and both our husbands. I dissolved into laughter.

Her eyes sparkled. "I thought a new dress would lift your spirits, so I searched every aisle of the Salvation Army store to find the right one. Don't you think it's perfect? It shouldn't feel too tight!"

Bob and Page were howling, too. "Well," I said between giggles, "I certainly don't have anything like it!"

At home, I considered my friend and all she did to encourage me and keep me lighthearted about a serious illness. Tonight she had cleverly made a point about my excessive complaining.

On the kitchen counter I saw her most recent card. She'd tucked a small magnet inside, and drawn a smiley face on the note she enclosed.

"...I commend you both for the caring, confident and courageous way you've gone ahead in your treatment. I know—as a

nurse—that your attitude will play a huge role in your healing..."
I already knew how important attitude was to my recovery. In the area of my weight, though, I'd slipped into a negative mode. Tonight Sandy made me realize I needed to change this.

I folded the dress carefully, then walked to the hall closet to tuck it safely away on the back of a shelf. When I needed a laugh, I would take it out and think of my good friend.

"Look For The Good"

"Be strong and of a good courage, fear not, nor be afraid."

Deuteronomy 31:6 (Scofield)

"Welcome back!" a chorus of young voices shouted as I entered the third and fourth grade classroom where Marion— my grandmotherly partner—and I taught Sunday School. I stopped in my tracks, caught off guard by this reception. Opposite the door, a brightly colored banner said, "Welcome Back, Mrs. Hackett."

"Wow!" I said in surprise. "I've only been gone four weeks."

Suddenly two girls rushed to hug me, their young hands warm and soothing against my neck.

"Your banner is wonderful," I said with delight. "You've worked hard to welcome me back."

Marion's eyes were shining. "The students planned it all. We've been worried about you."

"I don't know what to say, except thank you."

The other children were huddled around low wooden tables covered with sheets of construction paper, scissors and glue. Crayons and markers were scattered across the table tops.

144

"Don't look!" they cried as they covered their art work with their small hands.

Marian pulled me aside. "It's a surprise," she said softly. "We didn't expect you back so soon. They're making cards for you."

I shielded my eyes from them. "I won't look until you're finished."

The cards complete, I joined the children at the tables. Their faces glowed with more than Sunday scrubbings. "This is beautiful," I said as I opened each drawing of butterflies, flowers and hearts.

All morning the girls clung to me as though I was a favorite aunt who'd come for a visit. Even the boys, though hesitant to demonstrate devotion, hovered nearby.

"I can't get over it," I said to Marian. "You'd think I'd been away for a year."

"Four weeks seems long to a child, especially when some-one has been sick."

I swallowed a lump as I remembered a Bible passage where Christ spoke of ministering to others. The disciples were bewildered by the parable.

"When, Lord," they asked, "did we ever see you hungry and feed you, or thirsty and give you a drink? When did we ever see you sick or in prison, and visit you?"

"The King will reply," Jesus said, "whenever you did this for one of the least important of these brothers of mine, you did it for me!" (Matthew 25:37-40 GNB)

I realized Christ's commandment had been fulfilled in my own life these past four weeks. I'd been sick and was visited; hungry and fed. When I was thirsty, especially that first day in the hospital when pain rendered me helpless, others had offered me water. Thankfully, I hadn't been sentenced to prison, but I'd been absent from this classroom, and today I was welcomed back with love.

Tears of gratitude stung my eyes. I felt I'd done little to earn their love, but so many had shown compassion toward me.

While the students finished their lesson, I sat in silence on a small wooden chair, unable to voice the depth of my gratitude, except to God.

Thank you, Lord, for those who minister to me.

* * * * * * * * * *

Other "well-meaning souls," however, caused moments of distress. Bob and I were seated at the kitchen table, discussing some comments people had made regarding cancer. The comfortable, homey smell of simmering chili wafted through the room.

Bob's eyes flashed dark with anger. "Remember the woman who said you'll probably need to have your other breast removed some day?" He seemed astonished by her words. "What a foolish thing to say!"

"It was dumb," I said, shaking my head. "She surely didn't realize how that sounded."

Why had she made such a careless remark, I wondered? Of the thousands of women with breast cancer, only a tiny percentage required double mastectomies.

"That's as ridiculous as the man who said I wouldn't have any appetite and would have to force myself to eat! One look at my swollen waistline proves how wrong he is."

"It makes me mad when people say these things," Bob said in disgust.

I nodded. "Comments like these indicate most people have good hearts but very little knowledge of cancer. They probably know someone who couldn't eat during chemo and assumed that's true for everyone."

The chili needed stirring. I rose from my chair. "Dr. Andrews cautioned against comparing myself to other patients. That was good advice. If I listened to everyone and their absurd ideas about cancer, I'd be terrified!"

The conversation reminded me how I'd inadvertently learned of a comment made to Tammy about my impending death. She'd been so distraught by the remark, Gary rushed home from work to comfort his sobbing wife.

Bob squeezed my hand. "I'm not going to listen to anyone else. I'll just watch you and see how great you're doing and forget all their ridiculous words."

I hugged him. "Good plan."

Our conversation triggered my curiosity about a passage in the book of James. After dinner, I looked it up in my Good News Bible. The words were underlined.

"Listen to this, Honey," I said. Bob looked up from reading the newspaper. "'The tongue is like a fire...a world of wrong, occupying its place in our bodies and spreading evil through our whole being. It sets on fire the entire course of our existence...'"Bob listened as I continued reading. "'But no one has ever been able to tame the tongue. It is evil and uncontrollable, full of deadly poison.'

"That's strong language," I said, looking thoughtfully at my husband, "but I think good old James hit the nail right on the head. Careless words drive people apart more than anything else."

Convicted of my own shortcomings by the words I read, I rose from the couch and nestled my head against Bob's shoulder. "I'm sorry for all the foolish remarks I've made through the years. Will you forgive me?"

He hugged me. "Of course. I love you."

"I love you, too."

* * * * * * * * *

My lips pursed with reluctance, I pulled three small plastic medicine bottles from my purse and placed them on my tray in the faculty cafeteria next to my glass of milk.

Might as well wave a skull and crossbones, I thought.

No one in the circle around the table mentioned the pills. In fact, it was as if they had agreed to ignore them. I said nothing, either, but they must have guessed what the pills were for; I'd seldom taken medicine at lunchtime before. I wanted to keep the chemotherapy pills hidden inside my purse, but fear of forgetting to take them prevented my doing so.

Each day I fidgeted as I uncapped the bottles and downed the medicine, a daily trauma as I felt the pills reminded everyone at the table of the deadly cells within me. That was the last thing I wanted to have happen.

After weeks of this routine, I emptied the pills into my hand under the table, then swallowed them discreetly. Maybe no one else cared, but I did.

* * * * * * * * * *

Like everyone else in the midwest, I was eager for warm weather, but an April ice storm erased all hope of an early spring. Complaints at school about the gloomy, gray day and the problems the ice had created were ongoing. Even so, I set out that evening for a women's meeting at church. My saintly white-haired friend, Muriel, agreed to ride with me.

She slid onto the seat beside me. "Hasn't it been a beautiful day!" she exclaimed. Her hand swept in an arc toward the ice-encrusted tree branches and street lights. "Doesn't everything seem to glisten? I just love to look at it." Her voice was soft and filled with wonder, and her face glowed like the car lights shimmering on the ice. There was no mistaking her real delight in the scene around us.

It was Muriel's consistently positive attitude that endeared her to all who knew her. She was a constant source of inspiration, a rare women who wore a cloak of tranquility despite the early deaths of three of her five children. One beautiful daughter—her youngest—was a victim of cancer, while other illnesses claimed two older children. I often wondered how Muriel and her husband endured so much sorrow.

I stared at her in amazement now. "Everyone else complains about the weather, but you say it's beautiful."

She pursed her lips as though deep in thought, then smiled peacefully. "You have to look for the good," she said in a soft voice. "I learned that long ago."

"What an attitude," I said, shaking my head. "You're an absolute wonder, and I'm blessed to know you." I reached over to pat her hand.

"So much of life is what we make of it," Muriel said. Her blue eyes sparkled. There was a quiet conviction in her voice. "Harv and I have been through some sad times, but God has always been there with us. Knowing that kept us going."

Through the night and into the next day I pondered Muriel's words. "Look for the good," she said. Could good come from my cancer experience? Would cancer make me a stronger Christian, a less demanding wife? Would I someday look back on this difficult experience, as I had the black days in Batavia, and discover that good truly had come from this illness?

Perhaps. Even now, as I endeavored to demonstrate a positive attitude toward the disease, an incredible thing was happening. A casual conversation with someone experiencing problems or difficulty in a relationship would turn into a counseling session. I was so eager to share my confidence in God's power to restore and renew, I couldn't refrain from saying this to others. "Nothing is too great for God," I said. "Believe that He will help you through this. Don't be afraid to ask for His help. Then study yourself and your own strengths to see how you can make your situation better."

"And most of all," I added with a grin, "look for the good."

* * * * * * * * * *

At last I understood the significance of the estrogen-positive lump. It was to my benefit that I hadn't known its meaning sooner.

In layman's terms, "estrogen-positive" meant the lump had been fed from my body's estrogen. As a precaution against further estrogen-consuming lumps, chemotherapy had halted the production of this pituitary-based substance.

I hadn't known until now that estrogen was my body's moisturizing agent. Deprived of its natural lubricant, my cells craved moisture as if I'd run a marathon through the Sahara. All day I gulped water and chewed gum, never fully satisfying my thirst.

Nighttime was worse. I awoke often—my mouth dry as the stuffing in my pillow—driven from bed in search of water. The more I drank, the more trips I made to the bathroom.

I saw a difference in my skin, too, as it screamed for layers of lotion. My shiny, healthy hair was now lifeless and coarse.

The most remote parts of me demanded lubrication. In *Chemotherapy and You* I read, "Hormone changes can also result in dryness of vaginal tissue." I didn't need to read this sentence to know its truth.

"I'm sorry, Honey," I said one difficult night. "I hate what's happened to me." Tears stung my eyes.

"It's okay," Bob said tenderly. "We'll manage."

In fact, we were experiencing a new level of joy in our relationship. From the moment I'd first mentioned the biopsy, the stresses that buffeted our marriage had disappeared.

Sunday mornings, when the tensions of the week had melted away like dew beneath a warm sun, we expressed our desire for each other.

"You'll never know how much I love you," I whispered.

"I love you just as much," Bob said, his hand caressing my face. The bedroom was as still as a whisper. Our hearts, our souls and our bodies were bonded into one. Ripples of joy ran through me. I didn't know it was possible to be loved so fully. After nearly thirty years of marriage, Bob and I had fallen in love again.

My sister enjoyed our revived romance.

"Is Bob still pampering you all the time?" she wondered as we talked on the phone later.

I laughed enthusiastically. "He sure is! I can hardly believe the change in him." I was in the kitchen, peering through the window at a family of squirrels who chased up and down the oaks.

"When I came home from work yesterday, I discovered the

dining room table set with china, the good silver and crystal goblets. A bouquet of flowers was on the table, and soft music was playing in the background."

"No kidding!" Deliece exclaimed.

"While I made salads and baked the potatoes, Bob cooked steaks on the grill. Then," I paused for effect, "after dinner, he brewed coffee for us. He's never done that before!"

She was laughing now. "I wish I'd seen that."

"It was incredible! And that's not all. He's learning to do laundry and shop for groceries, too!"

"Wow!"

"He's so agreeable, I'm almost reluctant to ask for anything."

Deliece giggled. "But you do, of course."

"Of course. I know a good thing."

"Don't take advantage of him," she warned. "Good men are hard to find."

"I'm trying to be fair. The truth is, I'm different, too, and Bob is surely pleased with some of my changes."

"What do you mean?"

"Well, my body's changed, of course, and I'm always tired, and maybe this is all connected, but I'm no longer driven to participate in social and community events."

"That is a change for you," Deliece agreed. "You've always kept a busy schedule."

"Can you imagine how relieved Bob must be that I no longer meet him at the door with a suggestion to go to a movie, invite friends over, take a bike ride or go for a walk? I've known his frustration over this, but I felt such a need to taste life's excitement."

"So, you don't care anymore? Is that what you're saying?"

"That's right. I just don't care anymore."

It was amazing how cancer had changed both of us. At last I understood Bob's need to rest at the end of a stressful day. At last I saw the world through his eyes—a world that demanded and drained our energy. At last Bob could come home to a wife who required little of him.

Maybe that was why he was so happy.

* * * * * * * * *

I still had one social request for my husband.

"Honey," I said one evening while he was engrossed in television, "let's have a dinner party to celebrate our thirtieth anniversary."

His eyebrows arched in surprise. "Are you sure it won't be too much for you? You're always so tired."

"I'll be fine. We'll keep it simple. It seems like the right thing to do." I didn't say I'd already created the guest list.

"Okay," he said reluctantly.

We booked the party at a local supper club, one with a comfortable, relaxed look and a small band. Deliece and Dick, Terry and a friend from college, and eight other couples joined us. Bob and I both wore blue, a significant departure from his rule of never dressing like "twinkies." Any more changes, and I wouldn't recognize my husband.

Our guests smiled broadly as they watched us toast each other with sparkling grape juice. "I thank God for bringing us together," I said thickly.

Bob hugged my waist. "He did a good job, didn't he?"

"He sure did."

Two decorated cakes suddenly appeared, surprises from our guests.

"You have to feed each other," one friend insisted.

Bob's eyes shone. "Open wide," he said gleefully before stuffing a huge bite into my mouth. Cameras flashed around us.

"Your turn next!" I grabbed a piece of cake and shoved it between his teeth. "This is more fun than the first time!"

We exchanged knowing looks, proud to have proven our skeptics wrong. No one could object to this union that had lasted thirty years.

We presented a small plaque to each couple as a remembrance of the occasion, a quote from I Corinthians 13: "The greatest of these is love." On the back were the words, "Bob & Delores, 30 years."

As the room quieted, I heard the band play strains of *Secret Love*.

I nudged Bob. "They're playing our song."

"Really? I don't hear a thing."

I tugged at his sleeve. "Come on! Someone must have requested this for us."

He walked me to the dance floor and slipped his arm around my waist. My arm circled his neck. We moved easily to the familiar music.

"Once I had a secret love," I sang softly, "that lived within the heart of me."

Bob smiled and held me tighter. I was floating on a cloud of memory, snuggled close to my love in the movie theatre while Doris Day serenaded a whippoorwill.

My head fell against his cheek. How had thirty years passed so quickly? In my heart, I felt nineteen.

"You've made all my dreams come true," I whispered.

Bob squeezed my hand. "You're the best thing that ever happened to me."

"I hope so."

We spun around before drawing close for a deep bow. In my mind, I wore a strapless gown with layers of stiff net above three-inch heels. A fragrant gardenia rested on my wrist, a gift from my skinny, crew-cut Prince Charming.

"I love you, Darling," I said.

"I love you, too." We danced on and on, oblivious to our disappearing guests.

When at last we went to our car, laughter greeted us, along with tin cans trailing from the bumper and a sign in the rear window, "Hitched 30 (tough) years."

"You got that right!" Bob said with a laugh. I pretended hurt feelings, but nothing could spoil the joy of this night.

We drove home to the sound of cans clanging against the

concrete. Each passing car honked; we laughed and waved in return. There was magic all around us. I felt young and vibrant, as though I really was a teen again.

I leaned against the car watching Bob nail the sign to the garage wall. Yes, some years had been tough, with the budget stretched almost to breaking, and painful periods of loneliness and depression. Through it all, though, nothing had destroyed our love for each other.

I reached for my husband and wagged my finger in his face. "Thirty tough ones, huh? Well, you'd better hang on for thirty more, Buster, 'cause I'm just getting started!"

New Life, New Hope

"Be delighted with the Lord. Then he will give you all your heart's desires."

Psalm 37:4 LB

Lauren toddled down the driveway to meet us, one little hand held tightly in her mother's and the other thrust away from her side to maintain balance. With each uncertain step, her brown ringlets bounced up and down.

The sight of my daughter and granddaughter made me forget my exhaustion from the two-day trip to New York. I sprang from the car almost before Bob could stop, and ran to gather Lauren into my arms. "Look at you!" I cried. "You were a crawling baby when you visited Grandpa and me in March." She smiled shyly at me.

"Hasn't she grown?" Diana asked as she drew us into a hug. "She gets into everything!"

Bob approached with our bags, leaning close to Lauren and grinning at her. She squealed and patted his face. "Do I look funny?" he asked with a laugh.

"You look great," Diana exclaimed, circling his neck with her arms. "We're glad you're here."

"Me, too," Bob said with a sigh. "I'm beat."

"Let me help with the luggage," Diana offered. Bob gave up one bag to her.

"Poor guy," I said. "He drove all the way so I could rest."

Diana slid her arm through his as we neared the house. "You're the greatest, Pop."

An exaggerated frown darkened his face. "But why did you move out of the country?" He pointed to the wallet in his pocket. "I had to get my passport renewed."

"It's not that bad!"

"Almost," Bob said mischievously. "You're only two hours from Canada."

"Oh, come on!" she said, her eyes sparkling. "You could drive it in a day if you had to." She turned toward the house. "You're here now and you can nap all afternoon if you want. Come inside, and I'll fix you a cold drink." She appeared as happy to see us as I was to see her.

Watching her, with her quick speech, ebullient mannerisms and feisty disposition, was like an image of myself. "Say what you really mean," Bob had often teased, knowing she always did. She was like her father, too, gifted with compassion and wit.

We followed her into their Tudor style home with its black shutters and white siding. I quickly saw that everything inside was neat and clean.

My arm slipped around her waist. "I'm so happy to be in your lovely home. I miss you back in Moline."

"I miss you, too."

"I'm thankful you have good friends in Fairport, though.

That comforts me." We exchanged thoughtful looks.

"I remember the night you were born," I said brightly. "You looked like a tadpole with long arms and legs dangling from your tiny body!" I gazed at her again. "And your legs kept getting longer!"

"I know," she agreed. "But it's great being tall. I never get lost in a crowd!"

"I've always wished I was taller," I said longingly.

Diana flashed an impish grin. "You are pretty short."

"I may be short, but I'm mighty!" I said with determination.

Diana rolled her eyes. "We just let you think you are!"

She poured glasses of iced tea for us and set them on the table. Lauren squealed in her high chair as orange juice dribbled down her bib.

"Your life has changed a lot this year," I said to my daughter. Her face glowed. "And I love every minute of it."

"You don't miss life in the business world?"

"Not a bit. This is where I want to be."

"I'm glad. I felt that way, too, when you kids were young." I remembered my letter to the editor years before. Diana seemed to share my views, with her own modern twist.

Bob had been listening quietly. Suddenly Diana looked expectantly at him. "When you get rested, I need your help with something." Her eyes sparkled. "You'll love it. You can be outdoors and get some exercise after sitting in the car so long."

He looked suspiciously at her. "What is it?"

She rose to pour more tea, a warm smile lighting her face.

"Washing the upstairs windows. I can't do them by myself. You wouldn't mind, would you?"

Bob thought a few moments, his brow furrowed as if the decision required consideration. " Let's see if I understand this. I drove 770 miles to rest and play with Lauren, and instead I'm going to risk my neck washing windows. Is that right?"

"You got it!" Diana replied, her eyes shining.

Bob's face broke into a grin. "Of course I'll help. I'd love to. It sounds like fun."

The next day, while I chased Lauren as she tottered through the yard, Bob leaned an extension ladder against the house and climbed to the top. In one hand was a bucket of vinegar water and a sponge. A ragged towel draped from his shoulder. Diana watched expectantly from inside the upstairs window.

Minutes later I looked up to see Diana frown at Bob and point accusingly at the window. "You missed a spot," she said mischievously. " Right over there."

"Hey," he protested. "I worked hard on that."

Suddenly the window opened and she leaned out, a bucket in her hand. "If Dad doesn't do this right," she called to me, "I'll throw this water on him!"

He covered his face in mock terror. "When I fall off this ladder, you'll have to wash the windows by yourself!"

I was surprised to have my thoughts suddenly grow wistful. *How quickly the days in New York will pass, and then we must return home.* I choked down the lump in my throat. It was true that life repeats itself; Bob and I and our young children had moved from our families too, and they'd been lonely without us.

Through long letters—Dad's graced with tender, poetic lines, Deliece's alive with family news, mine a combination of both—we'd kept our lives connected. Every important event and holiday had brought us together, sometimes for a scant few hours. Bob and I were trying hard to stay close to our far-away children, too.

I breathed a quiet prayer. "Help us, Lord, to always show our love to each other."

Lauren led me to the back yard where a plastic swing hung invitingly from a tree limb. I lifted her into it and gave her a gentle push. Her childish giggle charged the summer air.

I reached to pinch her toes as she sailed back and forth. "Is this the fun part, Lauren?" I asked, quoting a favorite expression from the office. She giggled louder. On the next pass, I squeezed her fingers. The giggle turned into a squeal. Ripples of delight flooded me.

Yes, my precious granddaughter, this is the fun part. This is the magic moment I will dream of when I am away from you. This is the memory that will comfort me.

Again and again, the swing with its beloved passenger sailed by. Time had stopped; the long miles had evaporated; cancer cells had disappeared. Only joy and peace and contentment remained. *Thank you, Lord.*

We finished our play, then sought Diana and Bob, who were packing up their tools.

Diana smiled gratefully at Bob. "Thanks, Dad."

"We make a great team!" he said, beaming.

I watched them with a sense of joy and delight. This was another special event to remember.

* * * * * * * * *

The kitchen was fragrant with the aroma of steaming pancakes. A dozen candles blazed from the stack Diana placed on the table in front of Bob. "Happy birthday, Pop," she said as she bent down to hug him. "Is it 51 this year?"

"Fraid so," he murmured with a sigh. "I'm getting old."

"Never!" she cried.

I smiled at him from across the table. There were times, I agreed, when his gray hair and lined face made him appear older, but today he looked rested and young.

His face crinkled into a grin. "Thanks, Skeez. These look great." From her high chair, Lauren giggled and clapped her hands, her eyes wide at the sight of the flaming candles.

"This scene triggers many memories," I said, my thoughts turned to the past once more.

"I know," Diana agreed. "Remember how we kids always dragged ourselves from bed, our eyes half open, to sing Happy Birthday to each other at breakfast?" She squeezed Bob's arm, a long-ago look shining in her eyes. "It was incredible. No matter how hectic our schedules, we made time for birthday pancakes with candles."

"That's right," Bob said proudly. "And I'm the one who

originated the idea."

"It's a great idea," I said, "even if I was the one who made the pancakes!"

Kurt laughed beside me. "Isn't that what Moms are for?"

I shrugged. "I guess. It sure seems that way."

Diana smiled wistfully. "Thanks for a great idea, Dad. I'm glad we have this tradition to pass on to our children."

"I'm glad, too," he said.

"Me, three," Kurt said brightly. "I haven't had pancakes in ages!" We all laughed.

Diana gestured toward the dwindling candles. "Make a wish." Bob closed his eyes briefly. I squeezed my eyes to hold back tears, remembering Tevye in Fiddler on the Roof. Tradition had been important to him, and simple, caring traditions like this one, were important to me.

With an exaggerated flourish, Bob blew out the flames. He caught my eye and winked. I wondered what he wished for. That the joy of this moment—with his daughter, granddaughter, son-in-law and me—would last a lifetime?

That's what I wished for.

* * * * * * * * *

"You have such a positive attitude," Deanna said at lunch soon our return from New York. A group of friends had gathered at a restaurant, and since I was on "summer break," I was able to join them.

"Thanks," I replied. "I have a loving God, and He is in control of my life. I'm not afraid." I'd repeated these words so often the past three months they'd almost become routine.

"It's important to me that I convey a positive attitude," I added. "Not long ago I read a magazine article about a mastectomee who was so miserable, she believed her life was over." My voice began to rise. "I'm frustrated by this kind of negative reporting because stories like this frighten women and their families. My attitude is much different, but hers sells magazines."

"We're always told bad news," Kathy said, " but I like to hear something good once in awhile."

"That's what I say!" I agreed.

"Are you keeping a journal of your thoughts and experiences?" Darleen asked suddenly.

I looked up, surprised by her question. "No," I said thoughtfully, "I haven't."

"You should think about it," she urged. "Your positive attitude could be a help to others."

I swallowed a bite of roll. "Maybe. But then I'd have to go to New York and appear on Good Morning, America and travel all over the country, and I'm far too busy for that!" Everyone around the table laughed.

Days later, another friend, Carolyn, came for a cup of early morning coffee. Summer was my chance to enjoy friends, and I was making the most of it.

"You always seem to smile," she said midway through our moments of sharing.

I pushed a plate of cookies toward her. "Thanks," I said, "but that isn't always true. I have to fight off negative thoughts like everyone else. At times, I wonder how chemotherapy can possibly kill every cancer cell lurking within my body."

Her face suddenly clouded. "I suppose you could think that."

"When that happens, though," I said quickly, "I repeat these words, 'I have a great and powerful God who can overcome all cancer cells.' That really helps. And I remember the positive encouragement from my doctors. It's a waste of time to be negative."

Carolyn reached over to give my hand a light squeeze. "That's a great attitude," she said softly.

"Do you remember the words of Reinhold Niebuhr?" I asked suddenly.

Carolyn looked puzzled. "Here," I said, rising from my chair. "I'll get them. They're on a plaque in the hall. The poem is called 'The Serenity Prayer.'" I walked toward the hallway.

"Let me read this to you," I said when I returned. Carolyn listened expectantly.

"'Lord,'" I began, "'grant me the serenity to accept the things I cannot change, courage to change the things I can, and wisdom to know the difference.'" I handed her the plaque.

"That's beautiful," she said, a catch in her voice.

I sat at the table again. "I'm trying to adopt this prayer into my daily life. I don't have enough energy to fret over circumstances I can't change."

Carolyn looked intently at me. "You should keep a diary

166

and record the events of your life now."

"You're the second person to suggest that this week!" I said in surprise. "I'd never thought of it before. The only writing I've done is letters and notes. Maybe I should think more about this."

After Carolyn left, I pondered her words. Keep a record. It was a good suggestion. Would the seed that had been planted some day sprout?

* * * * * * * * *

All day I'd waited for the phone to ring. Tammy was past her due date to deliver the baby, and when we talked in midweek she said the doctor would probably induce labor today. At the sound of the jingling phone, I nearly tripped over a kitchen chair lunging for it.

Tammy's voice was soft and strained. "You have a new granddaughter," she said, "just forty-five minutes old."

A rush of joy pricked my arms and slid down my spine. "Oh, Honey," I cried, "that's wonderful news!"

Thank you, Lord.

I signaled to Bob and he hurried downstairs to the family room phone. "I'm so happy for you, Truffles," he enthused. The use of her pet name seemed appropriate today. Even in motherhood, a daughter is still her father's little girl.

"Does the baby look like me?" he asked, his lighthearted giggle dancing across the wire.

Tammy chuckled softly. "No, she looks like herself. She has

light brown hair, and she's beautiful. We've named her Amanda Leigh."

What an old, old name, I thought. Aloud I said, "That's very pretty, Honey." I'd expected a modern name, but later I would learn that many of Tammy and Gary's contemporaries were choosing "Amanda" for their babies, and that Amanda Lee was the name of my great, great, great grandmother.

Suddenly I realized I hadn't asked about my daughter. "How are you feeling, Honey? Did everything go okay?" I fully expected it had since her pregnancy was uneventful and she'd taught school during most of it.

"It was kinda rough, but I'll be fine when I get rested up." Weariness edged her voice.

Concern for my daughter tempered my enthusiasm. "Oh, Tammy, I'm sorry. Will you be all right until I arrive Monday?"

"We'll manage. Gary's here beside me, and his mom will come soon. I'm kinda sore, that's all." I was thankful Gary's parents had moved to Arizona and lived near them. Joyce would be good support.

"Let everyone else take care of you and Amanda," Bob said, his voice soft and tender. "Your mom will be there soon. And I'll practice singing lullabies until I come next weekend." Tammy laughed again.

"Try to rest now, Honey," I added. "I'll see you Monday. I love you."

"I love you, too, Mom and Dad."

I hung up the phone and flew down the stairs. "Isn't it fantastic?" I said. "Another little granddaughter!"

Bob scooped me into his arms. "It's great!" His eyes sparkled. "But I thought you were too young to be a grandmother. That's what you always say."

"Well," I said, my heart racing with euphoria, "I am too young, but that's okay. Besides, I said that before I had grandchildren. Now I know better. Being a grandmother is wonderful!" Bob laughed and hugged me again.

"Amanda Leigh," I repeated. A shiver of joy swept through me. "Thank you, God, for a precious new grandchild."

In the kitchen, I recorded my thoughts:

New babies bring forth so many emotions. What joy to know the long period of waiting is over and a precious new life has been added to our family.

What potential for goodness—perhaps even greatness—lies within this tiny baby? Oh, the awesome responsibility for her parents to teach her and care for her.

Never again will their lives be the same. From now on, every minute of each day this child will be dependent upon them. And every day from now on, they will know the joy of being a parent.

The joys would outweigh the responsibilities, and nothing in the world could be more thrilling today than the birth of Amanda Leigh.

* * * * * * * * *

Throughout her pregnancy, Tammy had said she wanted me to "come take care of the baby and me." I was thrilled to be wanted and needed, but lately, as my energy continually withered, I'd wondered about my ability to do so. Did I have enough strength to be caregiver, nanny and cook for the next two weeks? What if Amanda cried all night and I couldn't sleep? What if she cried all day and my nerves were frazzled? At best, she would require midnight and early morning feedings. Gary couldn't help much; he worked long hours. Waves of doubt spilled over me. Would this be too much to do?

In earlier weeks I'd speculated about the chemotherapy treatments during my stay, wondering what I would do if I was scheduled for an IV when the baby arrived. Dr. Andrews had offered to refer me to an oncologist in Phoenix, if needed. Now, calendar in hand, I counted out the weeks—two with medicine and two without—and was thrilled to discover the fourteen days I planned to be with Tammy would fall precisely between my scheduled appointments.

The sound of Bob stomping his feet jarred me from my thoughts. He sauntered toward me, the brown and white "#1 Grandpa" baseball cap Diana had given him after Lauren's birth askew on his head and pulled low over his eyes. His mouth twisted into a hideous shape—similar to the ugly woman on the get well card from Sandy back in March. He was bent over like an old man, with his jeans hiked up to his chest.

"Gimme a kiss," he slurred, his arms outstretched.

I ducked away. "Don't even think about it, you goofy Grandpa."

He edged closer, his twisted mouth even more exaggerated.

"Come on," he chided. "Just a little smooch to celebrate our new grandchild."

"Get away from me!" I laughed. "You look awful!"

He hung his head and sauntered away. "I guess you don't love me anymore." From the other room I heard, "Everybody needs a baby, that's why I'm in love with you, pretty baby, pretty baby."

I ran to catch up with him. "I still love you, Grandpa, even when you act silly." My arms slid around his neck.

"I love you, too, Grandma." Just as I leaned forward for a kiss, his mouth twisted crazily again.

"Oh, you're impossible," I cried.

"I know. But you love me."

* * * * * * * * * *

Through the dining room glass slider, I gazed across the back yard to the great limbs of the towering oaks. As usual, playful squirrels scrambled through their leafy branches, their chatter like monkeys yipping in the zoo.

The afternoon sun began its descent over the horizon, and my thoughts were embroiled in a similar decline. *Oh, Lord, I miss my children so.* Sixteen hundred miles separated us. At times it seemed as though my new granddaughter and her parents were on the moon.

Why couldn't we all be together in Illinois? What good was it to have a new grandchild, when she was light-years away?

I wanted so much to be part of her life. But how would I ever be able to delight in her delights, cheer her successes and applaud her singing or dancing or volleyball games? What opportunities would I have to teach and support her as she grew from infant to toddler and into adolescence? I was already missing much of Lauren's young life in New York. With the distance twice as great, my role in Amanda's development seemed even more remote. I turned away from the door as haunting questions racked my thoughts.

What about the cancer? Would chemotherapy really make me well? Would I live to watch Lauren and Amanda grow into adulthood? Would we enjoy the same loving relationships I had shared with my grandmother?

I prowled through the house, pausing to look at college pictures of our children arranged in a cluster on the dining room wall. Wasn't it just yesterday they'd been babies? Then teenagers? How had they grown up so quickly? I leaned heavily against the wall.

Lord, I prayed, *please bless our children and grandchildren. Show me how to be close to them.*

* * * * * * * * *

It was Sunday morning now. Outside the bedroom window, a brilliant sun filtered through the oak leaves to spatter the lawn with patches of gold. I stretched and breathed a deep, satisfying sigh. Yesterday's negative thoughts were gone, vanished like flower petals during a thunderstorm. Tomorrow would whisk me to my daughter and granddaughter. In this moment, lying next to Bob, the whole world seemed right.

After breakfast I fashioned a three-inch heart from white construction paper and wrote with pink marker, "It's a girl. Amanda Leigh." Bob grinned as I pinned the heart to my dress. I poked him in the chest with my finger. "It's better than a neon sign!" I said.

"Careful!" he said, pulling away. "I'm a two-time Grandpa now!"

"And I'm a feisty Grandma!"

At church, friends congratulated us with hugs. It was good to be reminded that even in the midst of cancer, joyous happenings could still occur.

In the quiet of the hour, I realized what I hadn't known before. I would be a part of Amanda's life because my role in her growth began years before when Tammy was born. As surely as Bob and I had guided and nurtured our daughter, Tammy would teach her daughter the values she learned from us. I was already seeing in Tammy and Gary an assimilation of the lifestyle and attitudes Bob and I possessed. Through generational love, I would influence little Amanda.

The paper heart on my dress had become my badge of honor, the greatest pleasure my daughter could offer me—her child to love and cherish.

And tomorrow I would be with them.

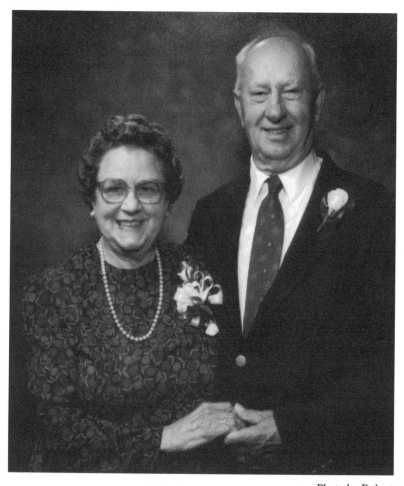

Photo by Robert

My stepmother and father, Dana and Lowell Woodall, 1991.

Strength in the Desert

"And thou shalt rejoice in every good thing which the
Lord thy God hath given thee."

Deuteronomy 26:11 KJV

The city of Phoenix and its surrounding towns sprawled
lazily across the desert like an overfed spider, its sand-caked
legs—with names like Mesa, Tempe, Scottsdale, Sun City,
Apache Junction, Gilbert and Chandler—creeping ever closer
to the red rock Mazatzal Mountains. Scenic forests and lakes
titled for an American Indian known as Tonto, a Spanish war-
rior called Montezuma, and a pale-faced, Harvard-educated his-
torian named William Hickling Prescott dotted the rugged
mountain range.

The history of the area mattered little to me. I only wanted
to reach Gary, Tammy and Amanda's home in Chandler, as
quickly as possible. It had been hard to leave Bob in Moline, but
his work required him to wait until week's end to join us.

The luxurious green of the midwestern summer was far from
me now, replaced by dwarfed and twisted sagebrush, wind-
tossed tumbleweed, darting lizards and slithering snakes. As our
altitude dropped, I saw stately hundred-year-old Saguaro cacti

standing guard across the barren desert like battalions of prickly telephone poles. Our pilot reported a temperature of 115 degrees awaiting us. Shimmers of heat rose from the tarmac to create an illusion of sun-drenched water. It seemed more than an apparition as the aircraft touched down, smooth as a paper boat on a pond. I hurried into the aisle.

Amanda, here I come!

* * * * * * * * * *

Gary dashed down the escalator toward the baggage carousel. I jumped from my chair to hurry to him. An hour had passed since my arrival.

We reached for each other's embrace. "Sorry you had to wait, Big Gal," he said, rolling his dark eyes. "We just got home from the hospital."

I smiled at Gary's nickname for me. Defining my tall husband as "Big Guy" made since, but me being 'Big Gal" bordered on the absurd. Even so, Gary always addressed us in this manner, a compromise between his preference of Mr. and Mrs. and our choice of Bob and Delores. I didn't mind. I knew his nicknames were spoken with love.

Gary grabbed my luggage and we pushed our way through throngs of people toward the exit. Keeping up with his long legs was a challenge. Outside, he said suddenly, "Tammy is in terrible shape."

My stomach lurched. "Oh, no!" I cried. "She said the delivery was difficult, but she sounded good when she called."

He shook his head. "She isn't good at all. She's in a lot of pain. She really needs you."

"Oh, Gary, I didn't realize." I grabbed his arm and ran beside him to the car.

In Mesa and Tempe, where Tammy and Gary had lived before purchasing a new home, stucco houses with yards of colored rock, palm trees, cactus and desert flowers had been the norm. The developer of this subdivision, however, must have had a longing for his eastern roots. All the homes were styled in a traditional Colonial design.

Along the sidewalk, rows of pink and white petunias thrust up blooms of welcome.

"They're beautiful!" I exclaimed to Gary. "It's hard to believe you can grow these gorgeous plants in such dry soil and merciless heat."

"I couldn't without the underground sprinkler system Dad and I installed," Gary said. He gestured toward the stretch of green that made up the front yard. "Digging in this hard dirt was like busting up concrete, so we rented a power trencher, and worked at night, when it was cool."

I could only imagine the difficulty of this project. The reward was this beautiful lawn before us.

Most homes in the Phoenix area were separated from their neighbors by six-foot stucco walls. Tammy and Gary's was no exception. I liked openness with one's neighbors, but the residents of Arizona seemed to prefer privacy. They also liked back-yard swimming pools, which would make fences a necessity.

Gary ushered me into the master bedroom. The drapes were drawn; a fan whirred softly overhead. Central air conditioning kept the house cool.

Tammy lay under a rumpled sheet. At the sound of our footsteps, she turned slowly toward us. Dark circles rimmed her brown eyes. I stepped closer to her side. *My poor baby*, I said silently around the hot salt in my throat.

"Thanks for coming, Mom," she said quietly. "I need your help more than I thought."

I kissed her forehead and stroked her chestnut hair. "I'm so glad to be here, Honey," I said eagerly. "But I'm sorry you don't feel well."

Gary had explained in the car that Tammy's cervical lining was torn by forceps used to deliver Amanda, but I hadn't realized the extent of her discomfort. By comparison, the births of my children had been wondrously easy.

"What can I do to help you, Sweetheart?" I settled on the edge of the bed. "Aunt Deliece is the nurse, not me."

"I don't know, Mom," Tammy said thoughtfully. "I guess I just need to rest while you take care of Amanda." She motioned toward a walnut cradle. In it, a tiny form lay wrapped in a pink blanket.

"Oh, Tammy, she's beautiful!" I cried as I turned toward my granddaughter.

"Thank you," Tammy said, a touch of satisfaction in her

voice. "I think so, too."

I knelt beside the cradle to reach cautiously toward Amanda. With my finger I traced the outline of her tiny nose and mouth, then leaned forward to kiss her wrinkled forehead. Her head was covered by a small, knitted cap. Despite the use of forceps, there were no marks on her perfectly shaped head and face.

"May I pick her up?" I asked hopefully.

"Of course," Tammy replied. Her eyes shone.

Gently I lifted the baby into my arms. "Amanda Leigh," I whispered, "this is your grandmother, and I've come to care for you and hold you close like this for the next two weeks. Is that all right with you?"

Except for the rapid pulsing in her chest, she lay motionless in my arms. Quiet sounds of breathing escaped her delicate nose. A shiver of joy rippled through me. Only hours before I'd been half a nation away; now I embraced my granddaughter. Tammy watched in silence, her expression a mixture of agony and pride.

My nose nuzzled against Amanda's. "Do you know how much I love you?" Her only reply was a deep sigh and shudder that joined the fibers of her heart to mine.

How privileged I am to care for this precious child! Even the dark threat of cancer could not deprive me of this special time with my daughter and granddaughter. For these first hours and weeks of Amanda's life, I would be her protector, and I would always try to shield her from harshness and pain.

For an instant, I wondered if God felt the same toward me. Did He long to hold me in His arms of love and shield me from the evil of the world? I wasn't submissive like this sleeping infant; I preferred doing things my own way. Maybe this was what Jesus meant when He talked about "being like a little child."

My eyes closed in prayer. "Thank you, Lord, for this beautiful child. Please keep her safe in your love."

The nursery at the end of the hall was furnished with a walnut-stained crib, changing table and matching rocker. *Perfect for Grandma and baby*, I thought as Amanda and I examined the room. A quick assessment assured me the cross-stitched quilt I'd completed days before Amanda's birth would fit the crib and match the room's decor.

Friends of Tammy's had given her a baby shower, and their gifts of stuffed animals, blankets, clothing and diapers were evident throughout the room. A bright paper border highlighted the walls.

"Your room is beautiful, just like you," I said to Amanda as we walked back to Tammy's bedroom.

Tammy watched as I eased Amanda into her cradle. "You have a precious daughter," I said. "I'm sorry her delivery was so difficult."

"She was worth every bit of pain," Tammy said, her voice strong with conviction. "I'd go through it all again."

I squeezed her hand. "But I wish you felt better."

Tammy grew silent. "I'll leave you alone," I said before tiptoeing into the hall and toward the guest room at the end. The bed had gone unused in March; it looked inviting now.

The sun was low beyond my window as I stretched across

the bedspread. A longing for Bob enfolded me; I'd never traveled this far without him before. At week's end, I'd be glad to have him beside me again.

He would be distressed, though, to see Tammy in such misery. I understood my children's concerns when they visited me in the hospital months earlier. Each of us wanted the other to be well.

And I was getting well, aided by chemotherapy and the faithful prayers of my family and friends. Scientific studies had recently revealed that prayer was a strong factor in healing. In Jesus' own desperate hours, He had demonstrated the importance of prayer. Earlier, He had instructed His disciples how to pray. Years later, the apostle Paul admonished others to "pray without ceasing."

All my life I had prayed for loved ones and those in need. Bob was also committed to prayer and early morning devotions. At mealtime we asked God's care over our children, and had faithfully prayed for Tammy and her baby.

Why she was suffering so now? Had we not prayed properly? Had God turned a deaf ear? Faith and doubt jabbed counter punches in my mind. I was convinced of God's healing power in my life, but He seemed to have overlooked our daughter.

I lay on the bed questioning, wondering and praying once more. At home, a basket held inspirational magazines and booklets. Among them was an index of 900 "pocket promises" from the Bible—many related to prayer. I believed those promises—God had answered countless prayers in my life.

The image of tiny Amanda, asleep in the walnut cradle next to Tammy, also drifted through my head. Tammy had labored to give her life—at the expense of her own body. But, my granddaughter was beautiful, every inch of her perfectly created like the rarest diamond in the womb of the earth.

Tears rushed to my eyes. *Now I see, Lord. You provided strength and courage to Tammy and preserved the perfection of Amanda.*

Our prayers for Tammy and Amanda had been answered by the presence of the Holy Spirit with them through the pain and struggle, the worry and fear.

I realized, too, how Bob and I had been comforted and connected to Tammy and this baby as we prayed for them. Prayer was as important to the one who prayed as those being held up in prayer. Through prayer, God had drawn us together.

A wave of thanksgiving washed over me. *Thank you, Lord, for your faithfulness.*

* * * * * * * * * *

"You need to make a list of things to do today," Tammy said the next morning while we shared breakfast at her bedside. "The most important thing is to take Amanda to the hospital to see about her jaundice. The doctor said to bring her in today for a blood test."

"But, Tammy," I protested, "I don't know where the hospital is."

"Don't worry, Mom, I'll draw you a map. You won't have any problems." Tammy was a master at making everything sound simple.

My face, hands and arms were covered with sweat as I dropped Amanda's diaper bag onto the floor of Tammy and Gary's car, then struggled to fasten my tiny passenger and her infant carrier into the seat. What did I know about baby seats and safety belts? My children had sat freely on the seat beside me when they were young.

Minutes later, wilted from the heat, I dashed into the hospital with my young charge. A woman at the desk directed us down the hall toward the lab. Poor, unsuspecting baby. In an instant, her blissful face erupted into a contorted, crimson explosion.

I paced round and round the room, rocking my granddaughter. At last, her sobs trailed off into a shuddering whimper. Grandmothering was not all joy, I was discovering.

Each day I drove the streets of Chandler with tiny Amanda in the seat behind me. Twice we returned to the hospital for blood checks; other days we visited the doctor's office.

Except for an occasional shuffle to the bathroom, Tammy remained in bed. Whenever I phoned her doctor, he was never available to see her, but his nurse assured me Tammy would soon feel better. The situation frustrated and frightened me, but with professional people instructing me to be patient, I tried to be. Tammy wasn't actually sick, I was reminded, she simply needed time to heal.

At last Tammy could sit up in bed. At breakfast, she began

her daily list once more. "First the grocery store, then the dry cleaner and the pharmacy," she said with a grin. "I think you can get back before Amanda wakes up."

"Yes, boss," I answered, tweaking her toe as it dangled from the edge of the bed. "I'll hurry, so I can come home and clean the house, do the laundry, bake the bread, milk the cows, mow the lawn, wash the windows and get ready for the ball!"

Tammy laughed. "Sounds good to me. While you're gone, I'll make a list for tomorrow."

"Oh, boy," I said, shaking my head as I walked away. The truth was, I felt thrilled to help, amazed at my endless energy. Was this the same woman who, for months, had been exhausted?

When the errands and chores were completed and Amanda was asleep in the walnut cradle, I stretched contentedly across the end of Tammy's bed. The afternoon sun cast hot beams into her room. Above us, the ceiling fan hummed softly, its blades turning ceaselessly. *Like parenting*, I thought. Neither ever stops.

Tammy was refreshed from her shower, her hair shiny and brushed. Pink blush brightened her tan face. "I hope I've taught you to be a good parent," I said thoughtfully. "I'd consider myself a failure if I haven't."

Our eyes met. She smiled at me. "You have, Mom."

For a moment, my mind was in the past. "Thanks, Honey. I seem to only remember my mistakes." She turned quietly on the bed, saying nothing.

"In the last few months," I said, "I've become more aware of the uncertainty of life and the importance of each day. I don't want to waste a single minute." I reached to squeeze her hand. I hope you won't, either." She listened in silence as though she truly cared about her mother's preaching.

"Remember the words of John Wesley?" I went on. "'Do all the good you can, in all the ways you can, as long as you ever can.'" Tammy nodded.

"Be the best wife you can, too," I continued. "I know this sounds old-fashioned, but it's worked for me. Gary loves you so much. Never take him for granted." Tammy eased cautiously to one elbow.

"And be the best parent you can. No one else is as important to Amanda as you."

I rose from the bed, bent over Tammy and kissed her head. "As for being the best teacher and daughter you can be, you already are! I love you so much."

Tammy's eyes shone. "Thanks, Mom. I love you, too."

My daughter had heard similar language before. Bob and I had expressed phrases of love and praise to our children since they were babies, encouraging them in all their endeavors. Nothing I said today was new. But it wasn't possible to say "I love you" too often, was it?

* * * * * * * * *

Agony was etched across Tammy's face. Our attempt to help her shop for a dress for Amanda's baptism had ended abruptly after one hour. The bag by her bed contained the only dress she tried on.

While Tammy rested, Bob, who had arrived a few days earlier, talked softly with me in the living room. "I don't think you can go home like you planned," he said. "Tammy can't be left alone to care for Amanda."

"I know. I've been thinking the same thing."

"We'll talk to Gary about it tonight."

As I'd done most nights when Gary came home, I warmed his dinner and joined him at the kitchen table. These few minutes each evening had been our only time together.

"I'm so worried about Tammy," he said between bites. "Do you think you could stay longer, Big Gal?"

I laughed and hugged him. "Sure I can. Bob and I already discussed this. I'll call the airline tomorrow and change my ticket. I'm glad you want me."

* * * * * * * * * *

Gary's parents and three brothers sat next to Bob and me in the front of the church. Before us, Tammy, Gary and Amanda faced their minister, a handsome man who sported a moustache and gold-rimmed glasses. His clerical robe hung evenly above his polished black loafers.

From the hymnal, Pastor Bert read familiar phrases. I focused on crucial portions. "Do you...accept your duty and privilege to live...a life that becomes the gospel...that Amanda be brought up in the Christian faith...taught the Holy

Scriptures...and give reverent attendance to the private and public worship of God?"

"We do," Tammy and Gary said together.

Pastor Bert lifted Amanda into his arms, then dipped his hand into the water and gently placed his wet fingers on her head. "Amanda Leigh," he said softly, "I baptize you in the name of the Father, the Son and the Holy Spirit."

What a privilege to witness this special moment! I was grateful Tammy had insisted on this date so Bob and I could be present.

Pastor Bert then prayed that Amanda's life would reflect God's love, and that she would be a faithful follower of Christ. In my heart I echoed those words.

* * * * * * * * *

I eased the door shut and slipped outside, breathing deeply of the fresh, cool air. After Amanda's baptism Bob had gone home without me and I missed him already.

A brisk walk would brighten my spirits and help dispel the gloom that enveloped my thoughts. Those who saw me as a positive thinker would be surprised to know my early mornings often were clouded with disillusionment and self-doubt. Long ago, I'd learned the best antidote was to rise quickly and get involved in some "action," be it housework, phone calls, baking or letter writing—in later years, my secretarial job— anything to "work through" my negative thoughts. Sitting lazily with the morning newspaper and a cup of coffee had never been beneficial to me.

I plodded aimlessly, my thoughts centered on Tammy and her pain-wracked body. All our efforts to aid her healing—bed rest, daily Sitz baths and antibiotic cream, seemed to have accomplished little.

"Lord," I prayed as I walked, "I thank you for this beautiful morning. I know you are here with us, helping us, but I'm worried about Tammy. She isn't much better, and I need to go home and back to work soon, and what will she do then?"

A water sprinkler splattered the sidewalk in front of me; I stepped aside to avoid getting wet.

"I feel overwhelmed, Lord," I continued. "Please help me to trust you and believe You are in control, and that all of these concerns will work out for good. Thank you for your love."

Words from the apostle Paul drifted into my thoughts: "I can do all things through Christ who strengthens me." The phase, from a favorite scripture (Philippians 4:13) carried a reminder of confidence and hope.

I repeated the phrase, recalling the same verse from the *Good News Bible.* "I have the strength to face all conditions by the power that Christ gives me." In recent years I'd come to prefer this modern translation. A spurt of joy ran through me as I considered the significance of Paul's words.

Walking faster and lighter now, I alternated my own paraphrases of these verses. "Through Christ, I can do all things. By Christ's power, I can face all conditions."

I was chanting now, a cadence, as my swinging arms kept stride with my rapid footsteps. "I can do all things through Christ. Through Christ, I have the strength to face all conditions." My arms flew higher, my feet strode faster. Adrenaline flowed through me as sweat beaded my skin.

Paul's promise pounded within my chest. "I can do all things. I can face all things." Nothing would overcome me.

The weight of concern had evaporated. I walked in confidence of God's strength, believing Tammy would be well, and so would I. Surely God's healing power—coupled with strong medicines—would erase all cancer cells from me.

"I can face all conditions. I can do all things." These past four months had proven this truth. Despite chemotherapy and the changes it created, I was living a full life, trusting God to carry me through each momentous day.

Above me, the sky was radiant with light. A smile beamed across my face. I lifted my arms like a gymnast at the end of her routine and marched down the sidewalk, the knowledge that Christ would supply strength to Tammy and me blossoming like the glorious flowers along this desert avenue.

* * * * * * * * *

Bob grinned and pointed to the cabinet next to the sink. Three weeks was a long time to be gone from home, and I'd forgotten which drawer held the silverware.

Hours later I began to feel at ease in the house I loved; Bob had cleaned and polished it all.

I strolled to the piano in the living room and looked at pictures of my children and grandchildren. Yes, I missed them and always would, but this was my home, and I was glad to be in it again.

The Dove

"I have the strength to face all conditions by the power
that Christ gives me."

Philippians 4:13 GNB

"What is so rare as a day in July?" It was easy to paraphrase James Russell Lowell's famous words on this glorious summer day. The sky was so blue it reminded me of Colorado, with only an occasional trail of white from a jet plane streaked across it. The temperature was in the 80's; there was little humidity. On-the-job pressure was not allowed today.

A nearly perfect Saturday, except for Bob's obvious dark mood. He moved with slow deliberation, his shoulders sagging from some undisclosed weight. His face was downcast and grim. There had been no playful kidding or joking during breakfast.

In fact, he barely spoke at all. I hadn't a clue what was troubling him, but something clearly was. Maybe he was falling back into the old pattern of worry. Did this mean the happy, carefree days we'd shared since the mastectomy were ending?

During most of our marriage Bob had been a chronic worrier. "I don't have to worry," I'd often said to friends. "Bob worries enough for both of us."

Was he worried about me today? Rarely did he indicate that he was frightened for me, but sometimes I could see evidence of fear in his dark, expressive eyes. They were truly a window into his soul. If I were to be honest, he no doubt worried about my health a great deal.

Since the diagnosis of cancer, though, he had seemed more at ease with his job—or else he hid his worries well. The end-of-day explosions had ceased. When I asked his opinion, he just smiled. "If you're happy, I'm happy," he said, whether we were discussing new carpeting for the living room or which movie we should see on Saturday night. He always seemed to want what I wanted.

The ironic thing about this scenario was that I wanted what he wanted, and wasn't happy unless he was. Today, I wanted more than anything for him to be happy.

I stole glances through the window, watching him at work in the yard. The lush carpet of green with its neatly trimmed sidewalk and curb often earned Bob rave reviews from neighbors and guests. "Mowing the grass long is the secret," he said. That, I thought, and weed control, fertilizer, frequent watering and hours of loving care.

Perspiration dripped from his face. His T-shirt and low-slung jeans were dark with moisture.

"How about a cold drink?" I called through the screen door. He nodded and waved. I watched him lean his rake against the house, then walk slowly into the cool house. When I kissed him, his eyes were clouded with concern.

"Something is bothering you," I said gently, handing him a glass of iced tea. "Does it have anything to do with me?" I always assumed I was at fault when Bob was troubled, though he frequently assured me I was not.

He stared blankly at me, then eased into a kitchen chair. "I have so much on my mind," he said wearily, stirring sugar into the brown liquid. "If only I could have peace." The ice cubes made a clinking sound as they swirled round and round.

"Want to talk about it?" I ventured.

He shook his head. "No. There's nothing to talk about." He patted my hand and smiled the resigned smile I'd seen so often. For awhile we sat in silence at the table. Finally, the glass emptied, Bob headed outside again. I stared sadly after him.

My ironing board was stored in a closet in the basement. I went downstairs to iron a blouse, Bob's haunting words penetrating the silence of the family room. *If only I could have peace.* How often through the years had I prayed for this very thing for my burdened husband? An only child who was reared in dingy houses, upstairs apartments or with relatives or friends, he carried an enormous burden of guilt regarding his strained relationship with his parents, who had been deceased for years.

Hissing steam announced the readiness of my iron. I began with smooth, steady twists of the hot iron across the collar and yoke—the way Mother taught me—then pressed the sleeves and finally the body of the blouse.

A quiet, indefinable longing hung in the basement air. I knew insecurities, too, scarred by a deep desire for acceptance that could never be satisfied. "They shall seek peace, and there shall be none," the prophet Ezekiel had written. Yes, everyone coveted peace. World peace, family peace, inner peace. When people were asked to name their greatest desire, they invariably replied, "Peace." Why, then, was it so hard to obtain?

I put the iron away, then headed upstairs to the kitchen to fill the sink with warm, soapy water to launder a blouse that required special care. Shiny bubbles danced and floated before me, iridescent globes exploding into nothingness. Wistfully, I watched them burst. If only Bob's worries could vanish as easily as these beads of encircled air.

"Please Lord," I prayed softly, "fill Bob with your peace."

* * * * * * * * * *

Outside the open window, golden patches of sunlight filtered through the giant oaks onto Bob's manicured lawn. "It looks beautiful out there," I called, my nose pressed against the window screen. "Come in for dinner now. Everything's ready."

He turned toward me, his face suntanned and sad. "Okay. I'll be right in."

We always sat in our designated spots at the kitchen table, like heading for our favorite pew in church each week. I liked being at Bob's right. I'd heard years before that sitting to my husband's right signified a solid bond between us. Mine was the choice seat, I thought, because it faced the large double window overlooking the deck, the back lawn and ravine. I never tired of this picturesque view, often accented by squirrels chattering and chasing through the tree branches, and birds sailing to the wooden feeder Bob had mounted onto the deck railing.

We held hands during the prayer. "Thank you for this food," Bob said, "and bless it to our use. Please protect our children and granddaughters from harm. Amen."

Steam rose from our plates of spaghetti. Between bites, I glanced at my husband, who responded with a weary smile.

Through the window, restful shadows graced the green lawn. I was reminded of another summer evening when a young deer wandered into the back yard and paused briefly to nibble blades of grass. Its innocent beauty had halted my breath in my throat. Deer must be one of God's most beloved animals, I thought. Their grace and delicate beauty seemed unmatched by any other creature. Slowly then, the deer had strolled into the ravine as though called to a secret conclave deep among the trees.

Tonight, a bevy of chirping, scolding birds gathered at the feeder for their own dusky meeting. "Look at them!" I said to Bob. "They remind me of kids on a playground, jockeying for the best spot." He smiled thoughtfully. The birds, alarmed by harassing squirrels, darted in and out, their beaks filled with seed.

While I watched, a flawless grey-pink dove unlike any I'd seen before landed silently on the railing. The air was suddenly quiet, the other birds hushed by the presence of the new arrival. For long moments the only movement was the steady beating visible beneath the bird's royal breast. At last the dove stepped with cautious serenity to the opposite side of the feeder, then tipped its head and peered at Bob and me as if to be certain we saw it.

I stared as though in a trance, incapable of diverting my eyes from the magical bird. It's haunting beauty captured me, much like the mystical quality of the exquisite deer of the past. Time had stopped and nothing existed but Bob and me and the spectacular dove.

My heart pounded a rapid, intoxicating beat as I glanced at my husband. "Here's your dove of peace," I said softly.

He looked up in surprise, his gaze shifting toward the bird. "Maybe so," he said gravely.

After lingering brief moments on the railing, the feathered messenger lifted its wings and soared effortlessly into the evening sky ablaze with pink and gold.

* * * * * * * * *

I rocked gently in the wooden glider. The late evening temperature on the deck was near perfection, neither too hot or too cold. Billions of stars glistened against the velvet sky above. *This is my favorite place to be,* I thought for the thousandth time. *It's so peaceful here.*

Rocking in silence, I heard only the rustling of raccoons as they ambled through the ravine, and the steady creaking of the glider swaying back and forth. Inside the house, Bob had fallen asleep in the recliner, his weary mind at rest. Everything around me seemed at peace.

I couldn't quit thinking about the dove, how it watched us so intently through the window, determined that we see it in return. There was no mistaking it had come for a purpose. The bird was a messenger from God, I was sure of it.

The words of Catherine Marshall, well-known author, tugged at my thoughts. In her book, To Live Again, Mrs. Marshall quoted from the sermons of her husband, Peter, a popular Washington, D.C. minister and Chaplain of the United States Senate until his untimely death at age forty-six. I stepped inside to locate the book in the bookcase.

"There are some things," Peter had said, "that can never be proven by argument, logic or reason; things that are matters of perception—not of proof. There are some things that can never be poured into the cold molds of human speech." Like her husband, Mrs. Marshall believed the Holy Spirit moves through our lives in ways we seldom recognize or suspect.

Returning to the glider, I pondered again the arrival of the captivating dove. A scene from the Bible came to mind, of Jesus standing in the Jordan River, his face shadowed by the outstretched hand of his cousin, John the Baptist. I remembered the familiar words. "And he saw the Spirit of God coming down like a dove and lighting on Him." (Matthew 3:16-17).

A shiver ran through me. The Spirit of God, descending like a dove. Now I was even more certain Bob and I had witnessed an event such as Catherine Marshall described. I had prayed for peace, and the answer had come, floating gently on the wings of the enchanting bird.

Since biblical times, the dove had been symbolic of peace and the Holy Spirit of God. I was reminded of Jesus' promise to His disciples: "I am leaving you with a gift, peace of mind and heart! And the peace I give isn't fragile like the world gives. So don't be troubled or afraid." John 14:27 (*The Living Bible*)

Surely those promises were meant for us today as much as when Jesus spoke them. I believed the beautiful dove was God's way of showing Himself to us and reminding us He was with us always.

I was equally certain the dove's message was two-fold, for Bob and me, separately and together. God wanted Bob to know His peace, and He wanted me to have assurance I would be well. This exquisite creature had come that in the days and weeks ahead we would always have this moment to cling to — a defining moment — when God spoke to us in a profound, yet simple way.

Fireflies darted through the dusk of evening, their chartreuse beacons flashing signals of promise and hope. I trembled, prompted not by night air, but by my awareness of God's tremendous love.

Don't be troubled, the Lord had said. *Have peace of mind and heart.* I was at peace, with no fear of illness. God's dove assured me I needn't fear; God would be with me in all things. If only those who pitied me could understand.

Neither was I afraid to die. The prospect of death meant reunion with my mother and grandmother, and the inexpressible joy of being in the presence of God.

The hour was late. I rose from the glider and stepped inside. I would not forget this night.

Perhaps I would dream of a dove.

"He Leadeth Me"

"And be sure of this—that I am with you always,
even to the end of the world."

Matthew 28:20 LB

It was happening. The very thing I'd dreaded the worst. The consequence of chemotherapy I feared the most.

Nothing could stop it. Not the one-a-day vitamins and calcium pills I faithfully swallowed. Not the healthy food I ravenously consumed. Not my earnest prayers and pleas. Despite all my efforts to preserve them, my lovely chestnut curls were falling out.

I stood trembling in the bathroom, my hairbrush poised in midair, as brunette wisps fluttered like dried leaves to scatter across the sink, the counter and the floor.

"Oh, God," I moaned. A great lump formed in my throat.

Wasn't it enough that my breast was carved from my chest, and my body as weary as if I'd hitched Dad's plow to my back and dragged it across a clod-covered field? Or that my skin and mouth were as dry as if I was stranded in the Arizona desert in July without water? Enough that I could barely squeeze my pudgy body into my miserably snug skirts and slacks?

Must I give up my hair, too?

I'd noticed the first fine strands falling free while I was at Tammy and Gary's, and hastily gathered them from the bathroom floor, wrapped them in a tissue and stuffed them into the wastebasket. *Maybe I can pretend this hasn't happened.* I'd never thought I was a beautiful woman, but I believed I had beautiful hair. My "crowning glory," as Mother always said.

How could I go to work, or anywhere else, without my dark curls? Would Bob love me without my hair? That night I'd tossed for hours, tormented by visions of my bald head.

I was desperate to ask Dr. Andrews about my vanishing locks. "I had hoped I'd be one of the lucky ones who didn't lose much hair," I said, my lip trembling, "but it appears I'm not."

We were seated in the room where I received my chemotherapy treatments. After three months of appointments—twice each month—I was comfortable with the proceedings of this little room.

Dr. Andrews moved closer to my chair. "Let's have a look," he said. I leaned forward while he sifted my thinning strands between his fingers. "Yes," he agreed, "your scalp is bare in places, but it isn't all that bad."

"How much hair do you think I'll lose?" I asked abruptly.

He leaned back on his stool, his fingertips together in the shape of a steeple. "That's hard to say," he said evenly. "Hair loss often occurs during the first half of treatment, then usually tapers off."

"I hope you're right. I don't want to wear a wig."

Dr. Andrews smiled. "There are beautiful wigs available in local stores. I'm sure you could find one you like."

I shook my head. "But I want my own hair, not someone else's."

He nodded. "I understand. For now, though, I think your hair looks fine."

Years before, when " beehive" hair styles were in vogue, each week a beautician backcombed my locks into an elegant, bouffant mass of curls that rose inches above my head. I recalled that period of my life as the only time I ever felt truly glamorous. The fashion of long dresses did much to increase those feelings, no doubt. By week's end, however, my oily coif badly needed shampooing and a fresh set, so I plopped an inexpensive wig over my own hair.

The situation was vastly different now. A wig wouldn't be a temporary cover up; instead, it would be a replacement for what I'd lost.

"How can I have a crowning glory," I complained to Bob, "when all my glory's falling out?" He held me close.

"How about a bright pink hat?" he said with a grin.

My lip hung down in a pout. "It's not funny. My scalp is peeking through for everyone to see!"

My "crown"—what was left of it—hung lifeless and limp. The rich, natural oil of the past was depleted; the strands were wilted and dry. Even with pink plastic curlers (saved from the beehive days), thick globs of setting gel and an extra half-hour of effort each morning, the daily rite of shampoo, blow-dry and style seemed a waste of time. Each day I headed off to work, attempting to convince myself my coif was acceptable. By mid-morning, the sight of my dull, droopy hair in the bathroom mirror made me want to cry.

Hopefully, Rhonda, the beautician who had cut and styled my tresses for years, could help. She was close to the age of my daughters, with broad shoulders under her protective jacket and long, thick, dark hair (I noticed it more now). We'd developed such a close relationship, Rhonda laughingly called me "Mom" when we discussed her personal life.

"Help!" I cried as I slid onto her salon chair. "I need you to save my scalp, and that's more than a figure of speech!"

Rhonda ran her fingers through my anemic strands. "You don't look as bad as you think. Your hair just needs some help." Her words reminded me of Charlie Brown and Linus as they stared forlornly at their wilted Christmas tree. Magically, their tree had become beautiful. It didn't seem possible Rhonda could create a similar transformation for me.

"I'll be right back," she said as she disappeared into the hall. Minutes later she returned, her arms laden with plastic squeeze tubes and aerosol bottles. "This brown goop smells bad," she said about one product, "but it will provide extra protein to your scalp and put life back into your hair." She explained that the other containers were filled with body-building mousse and vitalizing gel. "These products should make a difference," she added with confidence.

"You really think so?"

"I'm sure of it." She sounded so sure, but I harbored doubts.

"What happens if all this doesn't work? Do you think I'll need to wear a wig?"

She smiled again. "Hopefully not. But if you do, there's a shop across the river in Davenport that sells nice wigs. They're made of real hair, and look natural and pretty. Don't do anything, though, until your next appointment and we'll see how you look then."

I left Rhonda with renewed hope. Maybe she was right about me not losing all my hair. Her optimism reminded me of that night at Tammy and Gary's when I first discovered my hair coming out. I'd tossed for hours, sleeping fitfully, as images of floating hair drifted through my dreams. Music tumbled with me, an old Sunday-school song I'd learned as a child and hadn't sung in years.

He leadeth me, O blessed thought,
O words with heavenly comfort fraught. Whate'er
I do, where'er I be, still 'tis God's hand that leadeth me.

Over and over the comforting words rang through my head. Surely the memory of them was more than coincidental. I'd been certain God was reminding me of His constant presence in my life and that I should rely on Him to care for my hair.

Now, as I drove home from the salon, I hoped against all hope that the protein goop and gels and mousse on the seat beside me would bring new life to my tortured hair. I would try hard to focus on Rhonda's optimism, and trust my tresses to God. He was leading me.

* * * * * * * * * *

Terry and Anne had driven to Moline for a short break from their summer jobs and a few days of Mom's home cooking. I was clearing luncheon dishes and stacking them in the dishwasher when Terry strolled into the kitchen, his swim suit and beach towel draped across his arm.

"Anne and I are going to the pool," he said with an inviting smile. "Why don't you come, too?"

I looked up as I rinsed the last plate. "Oh, I don't know. I haven't been swimming since you kids grew up." I reached for the dishwasher soap and poured it into the cup in the door.

"That doesn't matter. We want you to be with us. It'll be fun. We can catch some 'rays' and go down the water slide."

I remembered my brand-new red and white swimsuit hanging in the closet, as yet unworn. The bright colors and permanently-shaped bra had caught my eye while shopping one day, and when I'd tried it on, I didn't look at all flat on my left side. I'd thought I might need the suit in New York when we went out on Kurt and Diana's boat, but we had been too busy to go to the lake.

"Okay," I said suddenly, "I'll go."

In the bedroom, I pulled on the suit, then stuffed a pair of

Bob's rolled-up socks inside the empty cup. "I guess I'm ready," I said as we climbed into the back seat of the car. Anne joined Terry up front. Her two-piece white suit effectively showed off her dark tan. I watched to see if their expressions hinted at discomfort with my appearance, but I detected none.

At the pool, I spread out my towel near the edge while Terry and Anne jumped into the water. Just as I was beginning to relax, Terry suddenly appeared at my side. "Come down the giant slide with us!" he urged. Water pooled at his feet and dripped onto my towel. I rolled to my side to avoid getting wet.

"Don't you think I'm a bit old for that?" I asked. I looked around for someone else my age. "All the others on the slide are kids!"

"Come on!" Terry insisted. Anne had come out of the water and joined him in pulling me to my feet.

"All right," I said. "You'll probably drag me if I don't come willingly." With trepidation, I followed them to the slide. From the high ladder, I could see all across the park.

"Remember when I tried to do this in New York with Diana and Kurt years ago?" I said with a laugh.

Terry grinned. "How could I forget it? I'll never know how you managed to turn around and slide down backwards!"

"I couldn't help it," I said, gesturing with my arms. "Every time I rounded a sharp turn, I spun around." The memory was vivid. My elbows had turned purple from bumping the vinyl edges of the slide.

Terry laughed and winked at me. "Try to face forward this time."

"Believe me, I tried before!"

At last it was my turn to go down. I stepped gingerly onto the platform. A college-age attendant handed me a rubber mat. I dropped onto it and slid into a swirling, descending stream. First one turn, then the next.

Suddenly I was underwater. When I bobbed to the surface, Terry and Anne stood nearby. Their faces were alive with laughter.

"Good job, Mom!" Terry cried.

"Yay," I sputtered. "I did it right." I stood up and headed for the side of the pool. At last I could rest on my towel in the sun.

"Ready to go again?" Terry asked quickly.

"Again? You said once."

"Well, he meant once, then twice," Anne said with a laugh. She was having fun with this, too.

Again I followed them to the top of the slide. Again I managed the quick trip down without twisting backward or smashing my elbows.

"That's my quota," I said as I mopped water from my face. "It was fun, but twice is enough. I'll sit and watch you."

"Okay," Terry said. I climbed from the pool as he and Anne swam away.

When I stood up, I discovered Bob's socks were missing from the empty cup of my suit. How could I have been so stupid? Nothing stays in place when it's submerged in water. In my haste to join Terry and Anne for a summertime outing I hadn't considered this fact. I looked all around in the shallow water; no dark shapes were visible. My hollow breast cup maintained its original contoured shape, but underneath the empty cone I was naked and disfigured. I felt foolish and betrayed. How could I have been so dumb as to rely on this crude measure to appear normal?

I hurried toward my towel and lay down across it, but the wet suit didn't cling tightly as it had before. With each movement, the fabric pulled away to expose my flat chest and scar. A wisp of cool air floated into the empty cup. I squirmed and tugged at my suit. Could others see my disfigurement? Did I look as bad as I feared?

Suddenly, I remembered Jane from Reach to Recovery, and her visit to me in the hospital. If only I'd followed her suggestions about swimsuits for mastectomy patients.

Terry and Anne joined me now, all laughter and smiles, eager to sun themselves on their towels. I lay unmoving on the towel, trapped in anguish, unable to tell them of my turmoil.

After what seemed an eternity, at last they were ready to leave. I wrapped my towel around my suit and followed them in silence to the parking lot and the security of our car. We drove past the elementary school Terry had attended years before. The red brick building hadn't changed much, but he was years older and more mature.

I was different, too, and the barrage of changes was wearing me down. I wondered what further changes lay ahead.

* * * * * * * * * *

My reflection in the dresser mirror stared back at me. I was a different woman now, grappling with the changes forced upon me. I wondered if I'd ever again change clothes in a locker room without self-consciousness, or sit beside a pool without fear of embarrassment? Would I ride my bike or take walks or play tennis without exhaustion? Would I ever be free of outrageous heat and its constant annoyance? Would I someday have thick, curly locks crowning my head?

In the living room bookcase I retrieved my copy of *Tested By Fire*, authored by Merrill and Virginia Womach. Merrill, a music salesman and professional singer, had survived a severe plane crash, but his face was burned away in the explosion. Years of reconstructive surgeries and painful healing had produced a new, unrecognizable face. Merrill wrote of trusting God to rebuild his life, along with his disfigured face. I was in need of a refresher from their book today.

"Nobody forgets my face," Merrill wrote. "That is a real advantage. Perhaps that is my way of rationalizing all the pain and suffering. But...to lock myself in a closet because people stare at me—would be to give up and die. Sure, there are bad times. I especially hate it when people look at me with pity in their eyes." (I could really relate to this.)

"I have a little conversation with myself at times like that. I say, don't feel sorry for me, buddy, I am alive and well. I have a wonderful business and I do what I like doing best. God has given me a song and I am singing it."

I returned the book to its spot on the shelf and walked back to the bedroom mirror. "Take a good look at yourself," I said. "Nothing has happened to your face. You've lost some hair, you weigh more than you want, and you get tired. But think how much worse things could be."

Something in the moment reminded me of Grandma. She liked to use a catchy phrase about "walking with the Lord." When I was young and heard her say that term, I thought it seemed old-fashioned and too evangelical. In Sunday School we'd sometimes sung a tune that began, "When we walk with the Lord..." Like "He leadeth me," this hymn wasn't sung much anymore.

The thought of walking or doing anything physical—with or without the Lord—was laughable. Tennis and bike riding were mere memories of past energy-laden days. Even if I had energy, summer was grinding down and my return to school was imminent. Then I'd be even more weary.

Still, Grandma's words kept rattling around in my head. I was, in fact, daily placing myself in the care of Jesus, depending on him to "walk" with me through the ups and downs of my cancer experience.

I remembered a scene from the Bible, of Cleopas and a companion walking disconsolately to the village of Emmaus three days after Jesus' death. When He quietly joined them, they didn't understand who He was. Later, as they ate, they joyfully recognized Him and their hope was restored.

So it would be for me. The Spirit of Christ was walking with me and giving me hope. Like Merrill after his near-fatal plane crash and the subsequent torture he endured, my life had more purpose than ever before.

I remembered the dove, too, sent by God to encourage Bob and me. "A defining moment," I called it, to hang onto when life looked bleak. A revelation from God to trust in Him.

Surely Jesus would reveal Himself more fully in the future as I endeavored to walk with Him. That was all I knew. That was all I needed to know.

* * * * * * * * * *

Menopause. What an awful word. I'd always thought women in menopause were older than me.

I first realized the truth of my new unwanted condition back in May when my menstrual cycle abruptly ceased. Without warning, the faithful, regular, every-28-days-nuisance failed to arrive. One month I was the same as I'd been for 37 years; the next I was an old woman incapable of bearing children. I didn't want more children, but I liked knowing I could still create them. The knowledge that I was capable of doing so made me feel young.

What next, God? I wondered. *I'm sick of all these changes.*

With the disappearance of my monthly cycle, another surprise developed. "You could have 'hot flashes' and other symptoms of menopause," I read in *Chemotherapy and You* as I

211

searched for an explanation to the surges of heat that coursed through my body. The word "could" made me laugh, as though hot flashes were a mere possibility rather than the continual blasting of heat and sweat that consumed me. There was no way to describe the discomfort that bombarded my body. I desperately wanted others to understand my misery, but no one could.

Dr. Spivey's comment in the hospital about the "estrogen-positive lump" surfaced in my thoughts. I'd dismissed his words at the time, assuming ignorance to be bliss. Now I wanted to understand the significance of the term.

"If the tumor depends on hormones for its growth," I learned from further reading in *Chemotherapy and You*, "hormone drugs can stop the tumor's growth." In other words, through the introduction of chemotherapy into my bloodstream, the estrogen hormone was eliminated from my body. There would be no more estrogen for further lumps to feed upon. Without estrogen, I'd been plunged full force into menopause.

Knowing the cause didn't relieve the discomfort. "I don't understand why my body thermostat sends all those 'heat up' messages to my brain," I complained to Bob as perspiration dripped down my chest and back. "One minute I'm totally comfortable, and the next I'm on fire and drenched in sweat." I wiped my hand across my slimy neck and extended a glistening palm toward him. "Look at this," I cried. "It's disgusting to be covered with sweat all the time!"

"Can I do anything to help?" he asked with a helpless expression.

I grabbed a towel to mop my face. "I don't know what. I'm so hot, I think I'll explode!"

I dashed to the kitchen to gulp cold water, clawing at the buttons on my blouse as I went. Feeling frantic, I yanked the blouse off and threw it to the floor. Next came my shoes and socks, then my jeans. Bob had followed me into the room and stood staring at me, stripped down to my underwear. He no doubt feared what I would do next.

"I'm melting," I said helplessly.

Distress filled his eyes. "I'll try to think of something," he said.

Weeks later, after repeated undressings and temperamental outbursts, Bob did, in fact, come to my rescue. "Your own personal cooling system," he announced one day as he retrieved three small electric fans from a shopping bag. His face glowed with delight. "You can station them around the house."

"What a great idea!" I cried. "Why didn't we think of this sooner?" With central air conditioning in the house, it hadn't occurred to me to operate fans, too. I threw my arms around my husband. "Thanks, Honey. These should give me some relief."

One fan was planted on the kitchen counter, where I stood blissfully in front of it (fully clothed), relishing the cool breeze.

The second fan went to a table in the family room, beside my favorite chair, and the third was carried to a corner of my desk at school. Throughout the sticky days of August, the hot flashes had seemed to intensify.

"Looks like that fan is in your pocket," I heard someone

say one day as I sat with the whirring blades inches from my face. I looked up to see a member of the Board of Education standing at the window, chuckling.

I laughed in returned. "Well," I said with a shrug, "it gets hot in here."

At first, I was self-conscious about the hot flashes at school. When someone was in my office, I tried to endure the inner flame in silence. But the heat quickly overcame everything else. Involuntarily I picked up a piece of paper and fanned it wildly, wiping my wet brow with one hand while the other tugged at my blouse collar. I couldn't concentrate on anything.

My body seemed to delight in playing tricks on me, because when I wasn't hot, I felt cold. This was especially true in later months as the weather outside grew cool. Gradually, I learned that the moments of coolness were merely a prelude to a gentle warming that suddenly burst into a blazing inferno. A dry-as-dirt throat was another hint of what was soon to come. Before the water could boil to brew a cup of tea to warm myself, a familiar tepid sensation began its trek across my neck and shoulders. Within seconds I was drenched in perspiration.

"Here I go again!" I yelled, reaching frantically for the range knob to turn off the flame. "Now I need ice water!" Having heard my outburst, Bob peeked cautiously around the corner.

"I'm sick of hot flashes!" I yelled, stomping my foot on the vinyl floor. "Sick, sick, sick!"

He sighed heavily. "I'm sorry."

"I know." I forced a smile. "This is just so frustrating!"

Within minutes, I reheated the water to warm my cold, wet body.

At my next appointment, I begged Dr. Andrews for relief. "These hot flashes are driving me crazy. It's horrible to be so uncomfortable all the time. Isn't there anything that will help?"

He shook his head. "I wish I could help, but I can't."

"Many of my friends take an estrogen supplement," I ventured hopefully. Actually, most of my close associates took artificial estrogen as a means to relieve hot flashes and control menopausal mood swings. I was envious of them and their comfort in church or at basketball games while I sat sweating and fanning furiously with the bulletin or sports program. "There's a draft in here," one friend chided mischievously. I hadn't realized I was making everyone around me cold, but I couldn't help myself.

Dr. Andrews looked away, avoiding my pleading gaze. "Artificial estrogen is available for women as they go through menopause, but, unfortunately, you cannot take it. It's vital that there be no estrogen in your body for future lumps to feed upon."

A sigh escaped my lips. "One friend read about medicines that don't contain estrogen, but still alleviate hot flashes. Could I take that?" I asked hopefully.

Dr. Andrews leaned back in his chair. "I don't recommend those drugs, either. Too often, the side effects create more problems than benefits." He stood up and patted my shoulder. "I'm sorry. I wish I could help."

We said goodbye, the matter seemingly having been settled. There was nothing I could do to reduce the heat.

At times, the fact my body had been forced into menopause made me melancholy and sad. Though I viewed myself as vigorous and vivacious, another irreversible change had occurred within me, taking from me the thing I most hated to relinquish—my youth.

Even so, I was determined that menopause and a mastectomy wouldn't make me old or less desirable. I draped my arms around Bob's neck one night and stretched up against his face. "I'm still young at heart," I said emphatically. "So bring on the frilly clothes and sexy perfume!"

Too Many Pounds

"Come to me all who labor and are heavy-laden, and I will give you rest."

Matthew 11:28 RSV

Bob's voice bellowed through the hallway and dining room, enroute to the kitchen where I was packing our styrofoam cooler with sandwiches, chips, fruit and soft drinks. "Hail to the orange, hail to the blue!" he sang as he high-stepped past me. I grinned at his impersonation of a University of Illinois drum major, his arms waving in a wide arc as though he held an imaginary baton.

"Hail Alma Mater, ever so true!" I chimed in as he marched by. We grinned at each other, then headed through the garage toward the car to load it for the Big Ten Conference football game later in the day. Bob squeezed a thermos of iced tea next to the cooler in the trunk, along with jackets, binoculars and stadium cushions.

Neither Bob or I could claim the university as our alma mater, but we'd grown up a few miles from the campus and always cheered for university teams. Before our move to northern Illinois, we often attended football games at Memorial Stadium and other special events at the domed Assembly Hall.

217

With Diana and Terry having selected the U. of I. for their edu-cations, our loyalty to the school was even stronger.

I hugged Bob. "We're going to have so much fun! A sell-out crowd of 70,000!" I glanced toward the blue sky above. "What a perfect day for football!" I handed him a container filled with chocolate chip cookies.

"Is that everything?" he asked, eyeing the packed trunk.

"I think so. Terry has the tickets. We'll meet Anne and him at the park for lunch. I guess we're ready. I can hardly wait!"

Bob shot a glance over his shoulder. I laughed. "You know how I love Big Ten football! It's so exciting when the band quick-steps across the field and the cheerleaders hurl their part-ners above their heads." I jumped off the ground, my arms raised above my head. "Rah, Yaaa, team!"

Bob grinned. "You're lucky we invited you. This is sup-posed to be a day for students and dads, you know. Do you look like a dad?"

"No, I look like a mom," I said impudently. "But you knew I couldn't stand it if you went without me. I'd have moped and pouted all week if you left me here by myself."

"I know. That's why we decided to let you come." Bob was laughing now. "You'd be worse than a little girl who didn't get to go to her first party."

I grabbed a cushion from the trunk and threw it at him. "You're not nice! The truth is, if you went without me you'd miss me." I swaggered up to him and gave him a kiss.

He giggled again. "You're right. I would. So come on, big

baby, let's go."

It was a three hour trip to Urbana, plenty of time to antici-pate the game, the Block "I" card section and its intricate pat-terns and slogans, and my favorite event, Chief Illiniwik—in ceremonial Native American clothing and headdress—creep-ing silently through the band at halftime before bursting onto the field to thunderous applause. I pictured him majestically dancing the length of the field, the fans entranced as he wove back and forth, his hands and arms held toward the sky as though praising the Great Spirit. Finally, he would stand solemnly while the crowd sang in hushed voices. A shiver of excitement raced down my spine as the miles hummed beneath our car. It would be fun, too, to stay overnight with Deliece and Dick. I was always lonesome for my sister.

Terry and Anne met us at a park near the stadium. "I'm starved, Mom," Terry said. "What did you bring? You know college food doesn't compare with yours!"

"Yeah, yeah, you're just buttering me up so you can eat lots." I pulled the sandwiches from the cooler. He reached for one. "I didn't have breakfast," he said sheepishly.

"How do you get along without me?" I asked with a shrug.

"It's not easy. You should come more often, especially with food!"

A sudden breeze blew our paper napkins off the table. Terry raced to retrieve them while I hugged my blue jacket tighter. Bob reached for his Illini sweatshirt and blue cap with an orange-colored "I" on top. I glanced at other parents and students who picnicked around us and realized our efforts to wear school colors were decidedly weak. Next year we'd have to do better.

"How about some shopping after lunch?" Terry suggested. "There are a few things I need."

"It's amazing how you always want to shop whenever we come to visit."

I winked at him. "Could it be that your dad's billfold is a little thicker than yours?"

Terry grinned. "Yeah, mine's pretty flat."

"We might as well shop," Bob agreed, "since the game is being televised and doesn't start until 7:00."

We soon discovered our family wasn't the only one browsing the campus stores. Everywhere we went, students were eagerly spending their parents' money.

I'd hoped today I'd be exempted from my battle with fatigue, but by the fourth store I realized this would be no different than all the other days when I arose fresh and eager, envisioning a possible game of tennis after work. As the day progressed, a neighborhood bike ride had more appeal. By mid-afternoon I was considering a brief walk on our street, and sadly, by quitting time I wanted only to rush home and collapse wearily onto the couch.

Now I lagged behind the others. Pain pulsed through my head, trailed across my shoulders and reverberated down my spine. My shoulders sagged as though they carried buckets of lead.

I staggered to the curb around the corner—safe from the traffic—as the others entered the store. If only I could hide out somewhere, swallow pain relievers and put a soothing heating pad behind my back. *What am I going to do? It'll be late when the game ends, and everyone will want to go for a snack afterward. Then there's the half-hour drive to Deliece and Dick's.* I breathed a heavy sigh. *How can I do all this?*

Minutes later, Anne, Terry and Bob joined me at the curb. "Looks like your mom has had enough shopping," Bob said.

I tried to smile. "I'm sorry, guys. I just can't take it like I used to."

The walk to Terry's fraternity house seemed 20 miles long. God, why didn't I stay home where I belonged? Why couldn't I be a contrite wife and let Bob have this day with his son without me complicating the situation? After months of exhaustion, I should have realized this day would be too strenuous for me.

We stood in line for the buffet dinner at the fraternity house; it appeared all the other families had arrived ahead of us. Pain raged through my legs and back.

When at last we were seated, I turned toward Anne. "Want to go to the game?" She'd admitted earlier that she wasn't a winner in the student lottery.

She looked up quickly. "Sure, I'd love to go. But I don't have a ticket."

"You can have mine," I said wearily. "I'm too tired to go."

"You're not going, Mom?" Terry asked, surprise in his voice. "When you love college football so much?" He sounded as though he didn't believe me.

"I know," I said thickly, "but I can't." I fumbled in my purse for the ticket. "It's okay. I'll watch the game on television with Deliece and Dick, resting in a big, soft chair. This way I can get to bed early." The image of the overstuffed chair momentarily soothed my pain.

Bob looked alarmed. His hand squeezed mine under the table. "Are you sure about this?"

"I'm sure," I insisted. "Besides, it's your special day, not mine." I handed the ticket to Anne before I changed my mind.

We agreed that I would drive our car to Deliece and Dick's, and Bob would drive Terry's car there after the game, then return it to him the next day on our way home.

Minutes later I stood alone in the parking lot outside the fraternity house watching Bob, Terry and Anne stroll happily across the wide lawn toward the stadium. They soon joined a throng of students and parents.

In the distance I heard the band as it marched toward the stadium. A voice boomed over the loudspeaker. I could see Bob talking excitedly to Terry and Anne; they laughed as though he had told a joke. He turned toward me and waved. Terry and Anne waved, too. My arm felt like concrete when I raised it to signal back to them. Then they melted into the crowd and out of sight.

Hot tears stung my eyes. It didn't seem possible to bear the sadness inside me.

I opened the car door and slid wearily onto the seat. My

forehead dropped against the steering wheel. "Little body," I said to the darkness, "you've always been so strong. Now you're a puny wreck. What am I going to do with you?"

* * * * * * * * * *

The smell of bacon drifted up the stairs and into the bedroom that formerly belonged to my nephew, Mark. Like my daughters, Mark was grown now, but in past years he and his sister, Laura, had enjoyed many happy hours with their cousins. Mark, who called me "Auntie," had chosen Terry to be Best Man at his wedding.

When I opened my eyes, I discovered I was alone in bed. Muted voices rose from the main level of the house. A glance at my watch revealed the hour was much later than my usual wake-up time.

I hurried downstairs, pulling my robe around me. "Hi, sleepyhead," Deliece said. "We thought you were going to stay in bed all day." She laughed and hugged me.

"I always have trouble getting out of bed at your house. Do you give me knock out drops?"

"No, I think you just relax more when you're here."

"Maybe."

It was heavenly to sleep late, but now I was behind schedule in preparing to go to breakfast at a restaurant with Bob and my parents before church. "Everyone else is finished in the bathroom," Deliece assured me. "It's all yours."

The warm shower was refreshing. Toweled off and partially dressed, I plugged in my hair dryer. I was already behind schedule and didn't want to be late meeting Dad and Dana, who were always prompt. I felt myself growing tense.

It didn't take long to dry my thin, limp hair. Creating an acceptable look from the scrawny tresses was the real challenge. I fumbled with the curling brush in a desperate attempt to make the lifeless strands presentable.

A sudden dry mouth and slight inner warming hinted of imminent combustion in my body. Those early sensations were quickly followed by the lighting of a blowtorch somewhere inside me.

I'd propped the bathroom door open to allow shower heat and steam to evaporate. Even so, the added moisture, elevated room temperature, concern over my hair—plus the knowledge I was running late—had no doubt affected my body temperature. *If I had a thermometer,* I thought, *the mercury would surely register 106.* What good was it to take a shower? I stood dripping wet again.

Frustration erupted like a geyser at Yellowstone Park. I thrust the door open and stood there, fiercely challenging anyone to come near. "I'm so hot!" I screamed.

Bob and Dick were in the adjoining family room, reading the morning newspaper. They both jumped to their feet. "I'll get a fan," Dick said as he raced out of the room. "There's one in the garage."

Bob dashed to my side and frantically waved the newspaper he held in his hand. He looked distressed, but a hint of a grin fought to burst through his sober expression. *He probably wants to say something funny*, I thought, *but doesn't dare.*

I shook my head at him. "I'm miserable," I said.

"We'll get you cooled down in a minute, Honey." Now he looked genuinely concerned. "I'm sorry you're so uncomfortable."

Deliece came to the door with a glass of cold water. I snatched it from her hand and drained it in one long gulp. Dick arrived with the electric fan. He plugged it in and set it on the floor beside me. I knelt down close to let the cold air blow into my face.

"Thanks, everyone," I said, choking back tears. "I'll be okay in a minute. All you Good Samaritans can go back to whatever you were doing."

I closed the door to separate them from me. Drying the salty moisture from my skin, I studied my reflection in the mirror above the sink. Nothing I saw—moist skin, pudgy waist, balding head—made me feel good. All my attempts to witness to others that cancer would not overcome, that I would win this difficult battle, seemed futile. I wasn't winning; I was losing the fight. I was trying the hardest I knew how, and it wasn't enough.

Outside this little room, my twin sister projected the image I desperately wanted to show. Hers was the cool, slim, energetic torso, her head crowned with shiny, thick hair. Mine was a caricature, a laughable joke the cancer devil had played on me.

I buried my face in my hands and dropped to the bathroom

floor. It no longer mattered whether we were late for breakfast, or if we went at all. I was desolate, longing for release from all the changes that cancer had brought to my life. "Oh, God," I whispered, "this is so hard. Please help me."

In the next room, I could hear the others talking and laughing. They couldn't understand how desperate were my thoughts.

I sat very still on the bathroom floor. The last remaining drops from the shower head splashed against the drain, then all was quiet. I counted the rows of squares that made up the design in the linoleum floor. Maybe I would stay in this spot all morning until I found the courage to leave.

"Come to me, all who labor and are heavy-laden, and I will give you rest." A calmness pressed itself upon me as the familiar, comforting words settled into my head. "Take my yoke upon you and learn of me. For my yoke is easy, and my burden is light."

Tears of release rushed to my eyes. "I'm coming, Lord, and giving this burden to you. Please bear it for me."

* * * * * * * * * *

I sat at my desk, staring blankly into space. Two school associates had recently died from cancer and a good friend was gravely ill. It wasn't easy to stay positive in the face of such knowledge.

Words that were framed in my mind during the morning prayer at church one Sunday now rang through my thoughts.

We don't need to know what is ahead
for us. We only need to live each day,
knowing God wants the best for us,
and that He loves us.

It had seemed certain in that quiet hour that God was speaking to me, renewing my hope and reminding me of His love. At the time, I'd hastily scribbled the words on the bulletin so I wouldn't forget. The memory of them now washed comfort over me like a warm shower.

Sadness for those who died and concern for my sick friend tore at me. *There's so much pain in life. Every day it seemed there was a new challenge to face.* Was it reasonable for me to expect to get well?

Something reminded me of a passage from Catherine Marshall's book, *A Closer Walk*, which I had recently read: "A Christian physician told me, 'I have seen an incredible difference in the patient's post-operative condition between those who saturate surgery with prayer and those who don't. They often escape sticky little complications and sail through the recovery.'"

Friends and family had supported me with prayer during my surgery and recovery, and I believed those prayers had made a difference. I closed my eyes to block out the sounds of students and faculty around me. *Lord, I need to hear stories of victory. Remind me You are still in control.*

I looked up to see Mike walk through the office door. He glanced quizzically at me.

"It's okay," I said. "Just talking to God for a minute. Now I'll get back to work."

"No problem," he said with a grin. "Say one for me, too."

I could easily say a prayer of thanksgiving for Mike. All through these months of chemotherapy he'd allowed me to be and do what I must, sometimes ducking out early when exhaustion overcame me or my appointment with the oncologist was scheduled during working hours. He hadn't indicated disapproval when he saw me writing personal thoughts on a tablet at my desk, even though my work was postponed for a few minutes. He seemed to understand the importance of getting those lines on paper as they came to mind.

He hadn't coddled me, either. My workload hadn't lessened; if anything, it had increased. By his attitude, Mike had helped me believe I was still capable of doing the job that gave my life purpose. I'd needed stability in my workplace, and I'd been granted it. Since that fateful March day, he had complied with my request for "no long faces." Never again had I seen pity in his eyes. He'd treated me the same as always. For that, most of all, I was grateful.

Now I took out a yellow lined tablet to write the thoughts swirling through my brain.

At the end of each storm, God sends a rainbow.

It's not the length of life that matters, but how that life is lived.

Each day is precious. I cannot waste a minute.

* * * * * * * * *

"We're moving back to Moline," Tammy phoned to say, the words rushing together from her animated voice. "The house is sold and the movers will be here next week."

That's wonderful!" I cried. "I can hardly believe it!" My heart felt as though it would burst with joy.

"Surely it must be God's will for them to move back," I said to Bob after the call ended. "How else could the details have all worked out so quickly?" He nodded. He didn't enthuse like me, but I knew he missed his children as much as I did.

I threw my arms around him. "I'm so happy! Why should we be sixteen hundred miles apart, when we could be in the same town enjoying each other?" I did a little dance around the room.

Thank you, Lord, for rainbows.

* * * * * * * * *

Weeks later Bob and I again drove the familiar stretch of I-74 to central Illinois. It was early morning. We were headed toward Carle Hospital where Dad was to have a Pacemaker implanted in his heart. High in the sky, a flock of geese soared above us, no doubt enroute to warmer air. There had been moments lately, like that day at Deliece's, when I had longed to escape, too.

As we traveled, my thoughts drifted to the past.

Deliece and I were always together. We played piano

duets. We sat next to each other on the school bus. We consoled each other if one of us was hurt.

I could never recall quarrels or anger between us, but there was an unspoken element of competition. Deliece had outdistanced me in high school just enough to be Salutatorian of our class, editor of the school newspaper and lead actress in the class play. "Ambition" was listed as her best quality in the yearbook; "Friendliness" had been ascribed to me. In the years since we had both enjoyed successes and joys in the workplace, as well as in our homes and families.

Personal appearance had always been important to both of us. It was especially satisfying, that no matter what our successes or lifestyles, we had continued to look as much alike after 49 years as any two people could. That was all changed now. I was still stinging from the memory of that difficult morning weeks before.

At the hospital, Dana, Bob, Deliece and I waited outside Dad's room for his return from surgery. "You keep complaining about your weight," Deliece said, "but I can't see any difference." She looked hard at my loosely fitted sweater vest.

"What you don't see is that I can't fasten any of my skirts or slacks," I said with a scowl. "Everything has to have elastic waists, and even then I've had to slash the waistbands to let them expand."

Near the nurse's station, Deliece spotted a hospital scale. "Step up here," she urged. "I'll weigh, too, and we'll see if there's much difference."

This is a bad move. The scales proved, as I feared, that my weight was ten pounds more than hers. "I told you," I said disgustedly.

"Oh, don't worry," she said. "You'll get rid of those pounds as soon as you finish the chemo."

I forced a smile. "I'd better." Except during pregnancy, I'd never before weighed this much.

On the way back to Moline that evening, I continued to wrestle with the matter of weight. Ten pounds would be insignificant to many, I knew, but I was a small woman, and I wanted to stay that way. I especially wanted to be as thin as my twin.

I didn't know how, but I was determined to lose weight before I saw her again.

* * * * * * * * *

At last I mustered enough energy to stroll along the Mississippi River with Bob. I was thrilled to be here after missing its beauty all summer. I looked into the sky above the water and I-74 bridge. It was a magical mix of blue and pink, swirled together like marbleized cotton candy.

Bob's arm curled around my shoulders. "It's been six months since my surgery," I said, lulled into reflective conversation by the deceptively calm water. At this evening hour, the water was so still and smooth it reflected the sky like blue-tinted glass. Underneath the quiet surface, though, a powerful current churned.

"You've come a long way, Honey," Bob said. " It hasn't been easy, but you almost have it licked."

"I've tried to maintain a status quo," I said, thinking of my job, the Sunday -school class I taught, our Sunday evening tennis with Sandy and Page, and my limited homemaking responsibilities.

"You've done great," Bob enthused, his hand squeezing my shoulders.

"It's discouraging because I'm so tired. I wish I had more energy." I looked wistfully at him.

"You'll soon be your old self again. Try to be patient."

We watched as a small dog ran past us, his owner chasing a dangling leash. We looked at each other and laughed. On the water near us, a gathering of ducks splashed and swam, and boaters enjoyed the fading minutes of daylight.

We strolled arm in arm along the long, winding asphalt path the parks department had created years before. Beds of flowers and memorial trees added to the beauty.

I turned toward Bob. "Sometimes I wonder what progress I'm making toward beating the cancer." He looked up quickly. "I mean, this isn't like having a bruise that heals or a cold that gets better. There's no way to know what's happening to the cancer cells." He pulled me closer, but didn't reply.

We walked in silence, drinking in the beauty of the evening sky. Shades of pink, violet and rose spread across the horizon. I leaned my head against my husband. The words from that meaningful Sunday worship buzzed again through my thoughts. *We don't need to know what is ahead for us. We only need to live each day, knowing God wants the best for us, and that He loves us.*

"Thanks for the reminder, Lord," I whispered.

Never Letting Go

"Love never gives up, and its faith, hope, and patience never fail."

I Corinthians 13:7 GNB

I leaned forward and twisted the volume knob on the car radio to better hear the Neil Diamond song that was playing. Traffic was steady on Moline's busiest thoroughfare. As the car crept along, I drank in the words to a song I hadn't heard before.

My devotion to Neil's throaty, sometimes offensive harshness surprised my son. "It's as though he sings from his soul to mine," I explained to Terry each time we discussed our differing opinions of the famous singer. "Especially his ballads about being lost and confused." Even now, with so much good around me, I easily revived the old hurts and feelings of rejection. Today's song, though, was about love. I listened more closely to the words.

"The story of my life is very plain to read. It starts the day you came, and ends the day you leave."

Behind and beneath and around the deep, distinctive voice, a glorious orchestral arrangement swelled and soared through the air like butterflies floating above a meadow pond. I was captivated by the sweet, haunting melody and unmistakable voice that delighted millions.

"It starts the day you came," the song repeated, " and ends the day you leave." Goose bumps covered my arms. The refrain perfectly described Bob and me. After thirty years together, I couldn't imagine life without him.

The romantic crooning of violins reminded me of a recent special moment as Bob and I prepared for bed. "Where's that lacy nightgown you used to wear?" he asked. "I'd rather see more of it and less of the high-necked old lady things you've worn all summer."

I grinned sheepishly. He was right in noticing the change. In spite of my earlier challenge to "bring on frilly clothes and sexy perfume," low cut, revealing gowns made me uncomfortable. They didn't seem proper for me anymore.

"The sexy gown is in the dresser drawer," I replied. "Maybe I should get it out again." And I had, and slid eagerly into my husband's open arms.

"I'll always love your body," he'd whispered, "no matter what."

"I'll always love your's, too."

Other romantic moments were of the experiences one reads about in novels. Over the course of the summer and fall, we had taken our place among great lovers like Romeo and Juliet, or Cinderella and the Prince. Bob's touch, always inviting, now electrified me. When he looked into my eyes, I saw traces of adoration.

"I love your cologne," he said. "You always smell so good."

"I love your kisses, all millions of them."

The Prince and Cinderella. I was resurrected from the cellar of irrelevance in the past to the stature of a princess in jewels and gowns. Though I did not look glamorous, Bob made me feel that I was. My whole persona was elevated by his devotion to me. He was, in every aspect of life, my Prince. And he proved his unwavering support each and every day.

"Would you like to go to Europe?" he asked after work one day. I turned in surprise to see an array of colorful travel books in his hands. "Or maybe Alaska?" he added with a broad smile. He thumbed through the pages, pointing out various tours while I stood speechless at the prospect of previously unfathomed vacations.

"Are you serious?" I finally asked. "Of course I'd love to see St. Peter's or the Alps. Can we afford it?"

"We'll find a way," he said with a grin. "I know you don't have enough energy for a big trip this year. Next year, though, we'll have a belated 30th anniversary celebration."

"How wonderful!" I cried as I threw my arms around his neck. "Let's do it!"

The traffic light was turning red in front of me. I eased the car to a stop as the Neil Diamond song lingered in the air. "It starts the day you came, and ends the day you leave."

Neither Bob nor I had ever left the other. I did consider it once, back in Batavia, but I couldn't leave my husband. Nor had he packed his bag to sleep in a hotel, although he'd threatened to leave when the stress of the job overtook him. I'd wept frightened tears. He had held me close and promised to stay.

Other images, equally unromantic, drifted through the brown sedan. Surely it was a miracle the kitchen cupboard doors hadn't fallen off from being slammed shut during difficult times. By the grace of God, however, we'd never said words too ugly to be forgiven.

I hummed another line from the song. "It's the story of our time, of never letting go..."

We had "never let go" of each other and the promises made on our wedding day. "For better or for worse, for richer or poorer, in sickness and in health, 'til death do us part." They were holy commitments, to be honored faithfully. Parting company had never really been an option.

As the car moved forward again, I thought back to our courtship years. Bob had written at least one letter each week from college during my senior year of high school. For a guy who played three sports, pledged a fraternity and held two part-time jobs, this was no small feat. I was romantic, too; all these years the letters were stored in a blue candy box on the closet shelf.

As I neared our home, I pressed the garage door opener and drove inside. In front of me hung the cardboard sign from our anniversary party. "Hitched Thirty (tough) years." I smiled. We'd faced many challenges together, but none any "tougher" than those of the past few months.

Once inside, I went directly to the closet to locate Bob's letters from college. I laughed at the cartoon drawings and nonsense comments in the margins, and the salutations of "Dear

Suga Pie," and "My Baby." Captured in memories, I reached for another box, one that held my letters to him. They were boring compared to his, except for the expressions of love throughout. How sure we'd been all those years before that God had meant us for each other.

The closet held other treasures as well. In my "Letter to the Editor" from years before, one sentence stood out. "I love my husband and want to provide him a home with tranquility and harmony." I smiled at this line. Though others might scoff at this attitude, it remained true for me.

The poem Bob wrote for the dedication of our home lay among the keepsakes. "A poor boy like me," a portion stated, "married a 'gal' too good to be true. In her Pollyanna way she never knew what it was to be blue....But all this could not be, without the One who sets us free. For the Hackett family would be full of strife, if we did not have Jesus at the center of our life."

Tears of joy sprang to my eyes. Everything in this past hour—the Neil Diamond song, the college letters, the letters to the editor and Bob's poem—had spoken of love, simple and pure. A tremor went through me, as though I'd touched an exposed electrical wire. Warm, glowing peace spread through my veins and arteries, my senses and nerves. Love was in the air I breathed, in the carpet and furniture and walls. Love from my adoring husband. Love from God whose love was greatest of all.

I sank quickly to the floor. "Thank you, Lord," I said softly, "for your love. Thank you for my loving husband, and all the blessings of our life."

I sat very still to absorb this wondrous moment. More words of praise formed on my lips, blended now with those of the 23rd Psalm. "You restoreth my soul. You comfort me with your rod and your staff. Even though I walk through this valley of the shadow of death, I will fear no evil, especially not the threat of cancer. For You are with me. You have prepared a banquet for me in the midst of this enemy. You have poured your oil of healing and love upon me. You have claimed me for your very own. You sent a dove to assure me. My cup of hope and goodness and mercy and grace and forgiveness overflows and spills into my very soul."

I took a deep breath and looked around. The room should have been glowing, but it wasn't. Only my heart and soul were lit by an inner glory. My words of praise were mixed with those of Paul in his letter to the Romans. "There is nothing in all creation—certainly not cancer or hot flashes or too-tight clothing or thin, straggly hair—that can separate me from your love."

Tears spilled from my eyes and rolled down my cheeks. "Thank you, Lord, for your loving, healing presence. Thank you for never letting go of me. For constantly pulling and prodding me to go forward in your power and love. Thank you, dear God, for giving me a loving husband to share my life."

* * * * * * * * * *

I quickly changed from school clothes into jeans—relieved to wear comfortable clothing again—then stuffed the washing machine with a load of laundry. It was a great convenience to have the utility room next to the kitchen where I could attend to laundry while preparing dinner. I smiled with satisfaction as the machine roared to life, then pulled the door shut between the two rooms to keep the noise level low.

While I cooked, the Neil Diamond song floated once more through my thoughts. *"And if I die today, I wanted you to know."*

Rarely did I consider the real possibility of death from cancer, but there were times, especially when I was tired, when doubts crept in. I suspected Bob feared the potential of death more than I. Our uncertain future was surely a great factor in the "second honeymoon" we enjoyed. Fear was a powerful motivator to change one's ways.

When the washer stopped, I transferred the wet clothing into the dryer and tossed in a scented fabric softener to help eliminate wrinkles.

Prayer eliminates wrinkles, too, I thought as I closed the dryer door and pressed the start button. All through our marriage, Bob and I had prayed daily for each other. Each morning as I prepared for work, I saw him in the living room, praying and reading a devotional. I was less disciplined, but I prayed often. Surely our prayers had lessened our fears.

And if I die today, I thought as I headed back into the kitchen, a lump swelling in my throat, *just wanted you to know how very much I love you and always will.* When he came home, I would tell him in person.

* * * * * * * * * *

The fall days were golden. At night, though, the temperature dropped considerably. For the first time in my life, I was glad to have cold weather; it was a great remedy for hot flashes.

I stood outside on the front porch in my shirt sleeves, breathing in the cool night air. "This is incredible," I said to myself. "I know it's cold, but it feels so good!" Above me, a crystal clear sky was alive with shimmering stars. I looked around in awe. For the few minutes I stood there, waiting to cool down, the cold and the beauty were exhilarating. I couldn't suppress a laugh. *Except for hot flashes,* I mused, *I'd miss all this wonder.*

* * * * * * * * * *

"We think there's an error in the report," the Medical Arts technician said, but it indicates your blood count is too low to tolerate the chemo today." She paused to allow her words to sink in. "Unfortunately," she continued, "we'll need another sample before we can continue." A cold chill went up my spine. I'm sorry," she said, sounding as though she really meant it.

"Me, too." The sight of her stricken face almost made me feel worse for her than myself. I forced a smile, then turned away from the sharp blade that slit my finger again. Silent words of praise to God helped distract me from this distasteful experience. When I looked back, the technician squeezed drops of blood onto three tiny plastic slides and spread them thin by rubbing matching slides across them. The blood quickly turned brown and dry before being spirited off to the lab. Thankfully, this second report proved me fit for treatment. I went off for my rendezvous with Alice.

She began by tying the tourniquet around my right arm and firmly tapping the back of my hand with her finger. The vein— which had puffed up appropriately each previous visit— remained alarmingly flat.

Creases formed in Alice's forehead. Again she patted my vein; again there was no response. I took a deep breath, then exhaled evenly. The lines in Alice's brow widened. Her lips were pursed with effort. "We may have trouble if we use this vein," she said, " but we need to try. I want to avoid your left arm if I can help it." I knew it was the policy of the staff not to administer treatment through the side of the mastectomy.

"Give it your best shot," I encouraged Alice, before realizing my pun. She grinned, then attempted again to inject medicine into the flat vein. "Ouch!" I cried, my body jerking involuntarily. "I don't think this will work."

She carefully pulled the needle from my hand. "We'll have to use your left arm," she said with a sigh. "I'm sorry. I'll try to keep from hurting you too much."

"I know you're doing your best."

Alice tapped the vein of my left arm and inserted a new needle. I tried not to move while the medicine traveled steadily up my arm and spread into my body, creating a warm, tingly sensation. At last the treatment was completed. I breathed a deep sigh. "I think that's enough cuts and needles for one day."

Alice's sweet smile caressed me. "So do I," she replied. "Things will surely go better the next time."

"I hope so."

Thank God, there's only one more time.

The Final Treatment

"I am come that they might have life,
and that they might have it more abundantly."

John 10:10 KJV

"No surprises!" I warned Bob as I shook my finger in his face. "Surprise parties are great fun for the planners, but the one being surprised misses all the excitement. I want the pleasure of looking forward to something special, so don't you dare surprise me on my fiftieth birthday!"

"Yes, Ma'am," he said emphatically. "You has spoken!"

I thrust my chin out in true Mammy Yokem fashion. "Remember what I said," I repeated, "no surprises!"

My birthday came and went, and there was no surprise. In fact, there was no celebration at all, other than the traditional birthday pancakes at Tammy and Gary's home. All week my feelings rose and fell like a roller coaster, disappointed there hadn't been a party, then hopeful one was yet to come.

Bob cautiously watched my actions and pouty face. "Your birthday won't be forgotten," he said at last. "Don't get upset because you haven't had a party."

By the Sunday following my birthday, I'd convinced

myself it didn't matter whether my birthday was celebrated or not. Turning fifty isn't anything to celebrate, anyway, I concluded. On the other hand, I was alive and recovering from cancer. More than six difficult, hopeful months had passed since the diagnosis. Surely this milestone birthday was worth celebrating. *So, when are we going to do it?* I wondered.

We finished playing tennis with Page and Sandy and walked together to the club parking lot, laughing and joking as we went. The tennis had been fun, but inside I was still brooding about the non-existent party, though I tried to avoid thinking about it since Bob had assured me we would eventually celebrate.

He opened the car door for me to climb in, but before I could, he reached into the back seat and pulled out a large brown grocery bag.

"What's this?" I asked guardedly.

"You don't have to wait any longer to celebrate your birthday," he said with a grin. Before I could say anything else, he plopped the bag over my head.

I was in darkness, unable to see anything. "How long do I have to wear this?" I asked, my surprise mixed with irritation.

"Just a little while," he replied, "so try to relax." With his assistance, I eased hesitantly onto the car seat and sat unmoving while he closed the door. In the background, I heard Page and Sandy's laughter.

Bob drove quickly to the street. Despite my efforts to follow the turns of the car, the bag on my head made it impossible to know which way we traveled. After several minutes, we slowed to a stop. Bob climbed out, then opened my door and helped me out.

"Surprise!" I heard as I pulled off the bag. When I could see, I discovered a large group of friends—Page and Sandy among them, as well as Tammy, Gary and Amanda—shouting and laughing all at once. "Happy Birthday!" they cried in unison. Behind them, a roaring fire lit up the night sky. I recognized the campfire site in a city park where we had picnicked in the past.

"Wow," I cried at the sight of so many people waiting for us. I wasn't angry anymore; I was overjoyed. "Where did all of you come from?" It was a dumb question, but all I could think of at the moment. Gary and Tammy's Sheltie dog, Irish, bounded from the crowd, jumping up and down and barking with excitement. I reached for him, but he darted away.

The others laughed and applauded. I looked gratefully at Bob. "You really did surprise me," I said. "This is terrific."

He put his arm around my waist. "Now will you quit worrying about your birthday?"

"No need to worry anymore!" I said with a laugh.

Off to the side, I spotted Dad and Dana. Their faces were beaming. A quick glance revealed that Deliece and Dick were not among the group. For a brief moment, sadness swept through me. She and I had talked on the phone on the actual date of our birthday, but after all the years of celebrating together, it seemed strange for her to not share this evening with me.

I knew she had celebrated with Dick and their friends and

relatives in Villa Grove, and Bob and I couldn't join them, either, so we were even. Sometimes, no matter how great the desire, the distance between us made being together impossible.

I rushed over now to hug my parents.

"Happy Birthday, Honey," Dad said. "We're glad we can help you celebrate."

"I'm so glad you came! Everything is wonderful! I can't believe it!"

Dana was laughing and talking all at once. "Bob and Tammy planned everything," she said with a sweep of her hand. I looked around to see colorful balloons hanging from the tree limbs and a brightly colored banner spread over a table.

"Nifty Fifty," I said with delight. "I hope that's true." The tables were festive with matching paper cloths and coordinated dinnerware. Hot dogs, baked beans, potato salad, cider and birthday cake covered the serving table.

I walked over to Tammy and took Amanda in my arms. She was wide-eyed at so much commotion. "Isn't this a great party, Amanda?" I asked. I turned toward Tammy. "I'm glad you didn't choose an "Over the Hill" theme!"

She nodded knowingly. "We knew better than to do that!

I hugged her. "This is great, Honey. You know how I love wiener roasts."

"That's why we did it, Mom, to make it special for you. Happy birthday!

"Thanks so much. It's a wonderful birthday!"

* * * * * * * * * *

"The air's so appetizin', and the landscape...is a pictur' that no painter has the colorin' to mock—when the frost is on the punkin and the fodder's in the shock."

The words of James Whitcomb Riley hung in the air on this glorious October day. They reminded me of the sights and smells of rural autumn, though I'd lived in the city thirty years and had grown more accustomed to its version of fall beauty in the trees that flourished along our streets and sprouted in the winding ravines.

I began the trip across town to the doctor's office earlier than usual. This spectacular fall day, offering opportunity to drive leisurely through side streets to soak up the day's splendor, was too glorious to ignore. I wasn't disappointed in my quest for color. On all sides, vibrant red and orange sugar maples greeted me, glistening in the brilliant sun like newly painted murals. Other maples glowed like amethyst and topaz jewels. Radiant burning bushes were lined along curbs and dotted across lawns. At each twist and turn I saw gorgeous colored leaves, sparkling and shimmering in the sun.

What a vivid contrast to the previous day when clouds had made similar leaves look dull and dim. "What a difference the sun makes," I said aloud. *And I'm the same,* I mused suddenly. Dull and dreary without God's love.

Today, however, no clouds dulled my life. I felt aglow like the trees. This was my big day—the final chemotherapy treatment. Soon there would be no more cuts to my fingers, no more needles in my veins. I would regain my energy and be free of doctors' appointments, or so I hoped.

I glanced at my watch and realized I'd better quit sight-seeing or I might miss the whole thing.

The lab technician, after pricking my finger for the final time and reporting healthy, rich blood cells, squeezed my hand. "Good luck," she said. "Take care of yourself."

"I'll try," I answered. A hush settled over us. We smiled at each other. "Thanks for all you've done for me." I turned and walked quickly to the patient room.

"Well, this is it," I cried enthusiastically. "I can't wait to be finished with this!"

"I know," Alice said, her voice dripping with sugary softness. She patted my arm. "Chemotherapy isn't fun, but you've survived very well."

"Thanks. I think so, too."

I watched Alice prepare for my treatment, aware how fond I'd grown of her during the past seven months. At each appointment we had chatted about our families and daily lives. I'd been one of her "ladies." She was always sympathetic about my hair loss and weight gain, and had studied medical journals in search of a means to alleviate the hot flashes. She had discovered nothing new, but I was grateful she had tried.

Alice spread out the equipment on the small table beside me. I sat quietly, studying her confident movements. As always, there were the vials of medicine, the tourniquet, the cotton swabs, the antiseptic gauze, the tiny needle and syringes.

Suddenly, I felt lightheaded. To steady myself, I took deep breaths and swallowed rapidly.

Alice swabbed the back of my hand and patted the vein to raise it under my skin. Then she gently nudged the little needle into the thin blue line. I shuddered as the liquid medicine flowed swiftly through my arm. "How does it feel?" she asked quietly.

"Like bubbles dancing in my vein." She smiled at my reply. "My stomach feels queasy, too, but I'll be okay."

"Take deep breaths," she instructed.

Oxygen filled my lungs. In minutes, my head seemed more clear. I smiled gratefully at this gentle, gracious nurse. She always had a soothing effect on me.

"I'll miss seeing you, Alice, but I'm so glad this is the end of these treatments!"

She nodded. "I know." In her eyes I saw a look of under-standing. She, more than anyone else, knew exactly what these seven months of treatment had meant to me. She knew every detail of the cuts and pricks and needle sticks. She had listened with compassion to my frustrations about weight gain, fatigue, hot flashes and hair loss. I marveled to think that every day, for eleven years, she had been instrumental in treating cancer patients like me.

Soon the syringes were empty and the little needle eased from my arm. Alice taped a cotton swab over the tiny opening.

It was over! I wanted to shout with joy. I wanted to grab

Alice and hug her and dance around the little room. If Dr. Andrews had suddenly come in the door, I might have thrown my arms around him, knocked his wire-rimmed glasses askew and kissed his fuzzy beard. My heart and lungs and brain were so electrified I felt as though I would burst. Every inch of me was filled with rejoicing.

I made no display of my feelings, however. Instead, I sat quietly on the chair and whispered a silent prayer. *Thank you, Lord. Together we made it!*

Alice gathered the supplies and tossed them into the waste can. As she walked from the room, Dr. Andrews did come through the door. Restraining myself from a joyous outburst, I merely smiled at him.

"Let's have a look at you," he said as he drew his stethoscope from beneath his jacket. I opened my blouse so he could listen to my back. "Deep breath and hold," he instructed. I breathed and held. "Deep breath again." Once more I complied. "Now exhale." He folded the stethoscope and tucked it into his jacket pocket. "Let's check the rest of you," he said as he turned his attention to my abdomen and right breast, my neck and arms, my legs and feet.

He rolled his small stool closer and sat down, facing me. His blue eyes seemed to sparkle. "I see no evidence of cancer in your body at this time," he said. My heart pounded in my chest. "I think you'll do very well."

I wanted to cry with joy. "That's wonderful news, Doctor!" I was amazed by my calm voice. It took all my determination to remain seated. "Thank you for everything you've done for me. I won't forget."

He smiled warmly. "Come back and see me in six months." We shook hands. I followed him through the door. Alice was making notes on a chart at the front desk. "Bye, Alice," I said. "I'm glad I got to know you, but I hope I never see you again!" We both laughed.

"I hope so, too."

"Thanks for everything." I turned away and walked out into the cool, clear October day.

My heart threatened to burst through my chest and soar into the magical autumn afternoon. Surely there had never been a more glorious day than this. *I'm free*, I wanted to shout. *I'm a free woman!* Free of chemicals and needles and razor cuts. Free of medical appointments and weigh-ins. Before long, I would surely be free of fatigue and weight gain and dry mouth and hair loss. I stood still, gazing at the magnificent autumn sky and vibrant trees around me.

"Thank you, Lord," I prayed, my eyes wide open. "Thank you for making me well. Please bless these people who have helped to heal me. I am so grateful for their care."

I walked to my car and opened the door. What I saw made me gasp. On the front seat lay a narrow green box. I reached for the tiny card attached. My hands trembled as I opened it. "To my beautiful wife," I read. "I love you. Bob." Tears blinded my eyes. I lifted the lid to the box. Inside lay a dozen long-stemmed red roses.

"Oh, Bob," I cried, "you're so good to me!"

The aroma of flowers filled the car. I buried my face in the roses while tears of gratitude trickled down on them. Shivers of joy rippled through my body.

"To my beautiful wife," I read again. With my hair thin, my waistline bulging and my skin coated with sweat, Bob knew I didn't feel beautiful, but he said I was.

I sat alone in the car, bathed in love from my husband. His love had been demonstrated often through the years, but never more tenderly than in this moment.

At last I started the engine and pulled into the street to drive home. Suddenly I burst into song. "Surely it is God who saves me." The words exploded from within me. "I will trust in Him and not be afraid. For the Lord is my stronghold and my sure defense, and He will be my Saviour."

More Than a Conqueror

"I will never fail you nor forsake you."

Hebrews 13:5 KJV

Mazie looked up expectantly as I breezed past her desk in the nurse's office at Moline High School. "This might be the day," I said hopefully. "My clothes don't feel tight, and when I tried on my green linen suit with a fitted waist, I could button it!" I hurried around the corner to her "official" scale, similar to the one I'd disliked in the hospital when Dad received his pacemaker. Quickly I pulled off my shoes.

"Good luck," Maizie called out.

For weeks I had stopped periodically at her office to check my progress at slimming down. I could weigh myself at home, but Maizie's scale was "professional" and therefore better trusted to be accurate. Each time I'd weighed at her office I hoped to read numbers that corresponded to my weight before surgery. So far, that hadn't happened.

Carefully I inched the metal weight across the bar. For a moment, I was afraid to breathe. Would I weigh more if my lungs were full? Within seconds, the weight hung balanced. This time, it registered the magic number.

"I did it!" I shouted as I jumped from the scale and danced back to Maizie. "I did it! I finally got rid of that extra weight!"

Mazie's gray eyes sparkled. "That's wonderful!" she exclaimed, laughing at my enthusiasm. "I knew you could do it."

I shook my head in wonder. "I had to. I had to do it, and I did!" I grabbed her hand and hopped up and down.

She grinned more broadly. "I'm proud of you. Many people never get rid of the weight they gain during chemotherapy."

"I know. I was worried I'd be like that, too. But, I did it!" Satisfaction and joy pulsed through me. "Now," I added, "maybe I can eat a few desserts."

"Sure you can," she agreed. "You deserve a reward."

Quickly I pulled on my shoes and hurried through the door into the hall. "Gotta get back to work," I said with a wave of my hand. "Thanks for the use of the scale. I'll see you at lunch." I paused to laugh. "Maybe I'll eat something gooey!"

She laughed with me. "See you later."

I was so excited, I nearly ran down the hall toward my office. *All that tuna and low-fat cottage cheese paid off*, I thought. I twirled through the door and plopped down at my desk. "Yes!" I said, pumping my fist. "With God's help, I did it!"

* * * * * * * * *

Would this miserable trip never end? At the wheel of the Oldsmobile sat Terry; Anne was on the seat beside him. Behind them, Tammy, Amanda and I were squeezed between the many necessities for a six-month-old baby, including the thermos of hot water to warm her bottle wedged between my feet. It was nearly impossible to shift my weight or stretch my legs.

Ahead of us in the caravan were Bob, Gary and their Sheltie dog, Irish, crowded into our beige Mazda.

The kitchen calendar back home featured a line of red ink and the words "New York" to indicate the week we all would spend with Diana, Kurt and Lauren to celebrate Christmas.

For fourteen tedious hours Amanda whimpered and cried, uncomfortable and unhappy in her infant seat. "My head is splitting," Tammy said as she tried unsuccessfully to calm her daughter.

The situation in the Mazda was also tense. Irish was nervous and stood all 770 miles with his nose inches from Bob's ear.

At last we collapsed into the welcoming arms of our daughter and son-in-law. It was exciting to see them, but we wanted only to find a place to sleep. "I have it all figured out," Diana explained. "Terry and Anne will be in the family room in sleeping bags. Mom and Dad, you're in the living room on the sofa bed. The rest of us will take the upstairs bedrooms." Irish would fend for himself, which meant he would sleep wherever he could find an empty spot—if he could.

All three bedrooms seemed somehow to be located above our couch; each footstep sounded inches away. Every kitchen noise and whispered voice drifted through the open doorway. The stairway was a mere ten feet from us; how many times can people go up and down steps while others are trying to sleep? Sleep, we quickly realized, was not the correct word for our situation.

"How are we going to stand this commotion for a week?" I whispered to Bob as we huddled under the comforter.

"I don't know," he said with a giggle. "It's pretty crazy."

The next morning I stared in dismay at what had formerly been a neat, attractive family room. Now I could barely see the carpet for the toys, books, shoes and boots scattered over it. In one corner was a stack of coats, blankets and pillows. Purses were piled in a heap near the adjoining bathroom, along with cosmetic cases, hair dryers and curling brushes. An infant seat and walker were poised to catch a careless foot. The scene reminded me of church camp, without the water balloons.

I tried to clear a path through the clutter, but the situation was beyond me. "I'm sorry we've destroyed your lovely home," I said to Diana.

"You haven't," she said brightly. "I love having you here."

I was assigned duties in the kitchen. "Honey," I said after three days, "you surely never guessed how much food eight adults could consume!"

"You're right," she agreed with a grin, "but we haven't run out yet."

I gave her a hug. "You're a terrific hostess!"

Bob had assumed the task of entertaining Lauren, romping with her on the floor—first a horse, next a tiger, then a clown. He crawled through the house behind her, making silly faces. "Come here, P.M." he said when at last he grew weary.

"Perpetual Motion" ran faster, giggling as she went.

"With Dad around," Tammy observed with a laugh, "who needs toys?"

When Lauren and Amanda fell asleep at night, the grown-ups sprawled on the floor by the fireplace to play Pictionary. Terry and Anne were master artists; Bob and I could barely draw stick figures. "Is this what you do at college these days?" I asked with an exaggerated frown.

Terry shrugged. "We can't study all the time."

I winked at Anne. "In the future, just watch television. I'm tired of getting beat."

At last it was Christmas Eve. A sense of magic in the air made it easy to forget the messy house and lack of sleep as I trudged with Bob and the others through freshly fallen snow toward Diana and Kurt's church. Each step made a crunching sound beneath our feet. The sidewalk and steps were ablaze with candle luminaries, while high above us, a Christmas star added its own radiant glow.

Inside, our family occupied one whole pew of the church. Bob took the aisle seat, with me beside him and Amanda asleep on my lap. When everyone was settled, I looked down the row at our family. A shiver of gratitude ran through me at the sight of us gathered together. I knew in that moment I would always remember this Christmas.

A parade of children filed past us, singing familiar Christmas carols as they went. It was fun to see them squirming in their holiday finery, their eyes shining like the sparkling lights on decorated trees around us. I leaned closer to Bob. "Diana helped plan this," I whispered. He nodded as though he remembered.

The room grew quiet as a handsome young couple walked slowly down the center aisle. Their clothing represented biblical times. A newborn son lay peacefully in his father's arms. When they reached the front of the church, Mary and Joseph knelt beside a wooden creche and gently placed their baby inside. Youthful shepherds and Wise Men quietly came from the side aisles to kneel beside them.

Baby Jesus. I looked at the baby on my lap. Baby Amanda. My eyes swam with tears.

The minister directed the congregation to stand and sing the closing hymn. With Amanda asleep in my arms, I stood with the others. Words to one of my favorite carols resounded through the church. "Joy to the World, the Lord is Come!" This great old hymn expressed man's boundless joy and praise for the greatest gift of all, God's son. I looked at Terry, seated next to Anne at the opposite end of the pew. He saw my glance and smiled knowingly. The anguished trip had been worth it, I thought, in order for us to be together in this holy place on this holy night.

"Let every heart prepare Him room..." God had been faithful to bring our family to this night of celebration. *Thank you, Lord, for this special night. I open my heart to you.*

* * * * * * * * * *

It was Christmas morning. Our bed had been restored to a couch, and the living room had nearly disappeared beneath the mountain of colored packages that surrounded Diana and Kurt's Christmas tree. A mixture of excitement and dismay surged through me as I pondered the scene. Within the hour, all this would be transformed into a sea of ripped-apart boxes, torn wrappings and bows, and piles of opened presents.

Why does it always end up this way? I wondered. How do we accumulate so many gifts? As the pile of gifts had grown, it was obvious we'd shopped plenty for Lauren and Amanda.

I was filled with gratitude, too. Back in March, when breast cancer became a part of my life, I wondered what this Christmas would bring. Now, here we were, our family intact, celebrating this joyous day together.

"Everyone who wants to open presents get in here," Diana called as she entered the room.

I'm ready!" I replied. The others wandered in, lounging expectantly on the sofa and overstuffed chairs. I melted onto a straight-backed chair next to Bob. Lauren ran through the room, giggling as she went, eager to help Kurt, Gary and Terry as they passed out gifts. Beside Tammy's chair, Amanda slept soundly in her infant seat.

Soon my feet were encased in packages. I picked one up and opened it. "Just what I wanted!" I cried. "My favorite perfume." I leaned over to hug Bob. "Thanks, Honey."

He burst into laughter when he unwrapped my gift. "You hauled these heavy fireplace accessories all the way to New

York, just so we can take them back home again?" He shook his head in disbelief.

"What else could I do?" I said, laughing. "I had to bring them for you to open on Christmas!"

In the midst of shredded wrappings and beautiful gifts, I saw Diana watching me from across the room. We winked at each other. Tears suddenly swam in my eyes. "I couldn't be any happier than I am right now," I said softly.

She nodded. "I know." For a while I was quiet, watching with contentment and sometimes amusement as each recipient acknowledged their perfect gift, knowing all the while it would later be exchanged for proper size or color, and duplicates returned. It was always this way, but money gifts were disdained in this family, as was the practice of drawing names. Each year we would fiercely shop for the perfect gift and hold our breaths to learn if it really was. Flawed though the system was, this was our tradition, and we would stay with what we did. We knew the importance of traditions.

The aroma of baking turkey drifted from the kitchen. "Smells good!" Terry cried. "When do we eat?"

"Hang on, little brother," Diana said. "We'll have it ready soon."

I rose from my chair. "I guess it's time to get to work. We don't want anyone to faint from hunger!" I stepped gingerly through the residue to follow my daughter to the kitchen.

When Tammy and Anne joined us, Diana began her instructions. "Mom, you're in charge of cooking the noodles and making gravy." She spoke as though she'd thought about this for days. I took the apron she held out to me.

"Sounds good to me," I agreed. "I'm sure I've had more practice making gravy than you girls have." Anne snickered behind me. "That's a safe bet," she said.

Diana turned toward Tammy. "You can mash the potatoes." Tammy nodded. "Fine. That's my specialty." Diana handed a sauce pan to Anne. "Cook the vegetables?" she asked hopefully.

"Sure. I can manage that."

Diana continued through the menu. "The jello is in the frig, and I'll bake the rolls Mom and I made yesterday." She glanced toward the oven. "Kurt can carve the turkey. I think that's everything, except filling the water glasses."

At last the dinner was ready. I was thrilled to see my daughter's dining table, impeccably set with her china, silver and crystal goblets. White linen napkins adorned each plate. Mother would be proud, I thought.

"Would you pray for us, Mom?" Diana asked when we were all seated.

"Of course." The room grew quiet. I bowed my head and closed my eyes. "Thank you, Lord, for this glorious Christmas day. Thank you for this food and happy gathering of our family. Most of all, thank you for Jesus, whose birthday we celebrate. Amen."

"And thank you for the Parker House rolls!" Terry cried heartily. "They look fantastic!" I chuckled under my breath. Parker House rolls and homemade noodles. Nothing else mattered as long as these specialties were served for Thanksgiving and Christmas dinners. The roll recipe had been Grandma's and was "labor intensive," as my daughters said, but the melt-in-your-mouth results were always worth the effort.

Terry bit into one now. "This is great," he murmured satisfactorily.

Diana beamed with delight. "Thanks, Terry." I felt a glow of satisfaction, too. Another tradition continued.

* * * * * * * * * *

"We won't be gone long," Tammy said to her husband as she pulled on her coat. Gary was watching a football game on television and gave no indication he heard her. The others lounged nearby, equally inattentive.

"We'll bring back Godiva chocolate," Diana promised, then quickly closed the door to the garage behind us. Outside, we laughed at the prospect of Gary and Kurt—with the aid of Bob, Terry and Anne—caring for the children while we exchanged gifts and shopped for after-Christmas bargains.

"I hope they realized we left," I said with a grin.

"As soon as someone cries, they'll know!" Tammy replied. We drove away before anyone could call for help, and minutes later, joined the hundreds who crammed the stores at the mall.

Our shopping completed, I begged for a break at Friendly's. I leaned against the wooden booth, gazing happily at my daughters. "It's great to have this time with you. We don't have many chances to be together without the distraction of the children or someone else." I reached across the table to squeeze their hands.

"It's a treat for us, too," Tammy said as the waitress delivered our desserts.

"I hate being apart as much as we have these past years," I continued, "but maybe that makes our time together more special."

"Maybe so," Diana agreed. "I love it each time you come. We always have fun together." She looked lovingly toward me.

Tammy nodded in agreement. "We do the best we can to be together, don't you think?"

"We try," I said wistfully, lost for a moment in reflective memories of past visits. Suddenly I thought of the enchanting dove from last summer. "I don't think I've shared with you what happened to Bob and me soon after Amanda was born." Both girls looked up.

"It was a Saturday, and your Dad was having a bad day. As usual, he wouldn't say what was wrong, but he moped around all day." I paused to take a bite of ice cream. "That evening, during dinner, a beautiful dove flew to the deck railing. It sat at the feeder and looked at us through the window. There was something so unique about the bird, I couldn't take my eyes off it." A chill went through me as I remembered the scene. "Ever since, I've felt God sent the dove to remind us of His love."

"Thanks for telling us," Tammy said quietly. "That must have been a special time."

"It was. Whenever things have been tough this year, it's helped me to remember the dove."

I was startled to see the waitress placing our check on the table. Was this a signal for us to leave? I wasn't ready for this lovely time to end; it seemed to have just begun. When next could we steal away from our responsibilities to enjoy ice cream and mother-daughter chit-chat? I looked at my daughters.

While we are together I must absorb each smile, each gesture, each hug. These would be the memories that would comfort me when we were apart. Ignoring the check, we talked and laughed until concern for our families forced us home.

* * * * * * * * * *

It was New Year's Eve in Moline. We had survived the trip home without incident. With Terry and Anne out for the evening with friends, and Tammy, Gary and Amanda back in their own home, Bob and I were alone in our quiet house. After our big week, quiet was nice.

Using his new brass tools, Bob built a fire that crackled in the brick fireplace. We snuggled contentedly on the couch, a bowl of popcorn and soft drinks on the table beside us. The television was alive with end-of-year festivities.

On this last night of the year, my thoughts turned to the past incredible nine months. Since the startling discovery of breast cancer back in March, I'd given up my breast and endured a seven-month trauma of chemotherapy. More importantly, I was alive, a "picture of health," my life almost normal again. At the conclusion of my treatments in October, Dr. Andrews had said I was "cancer free."

Even so, the experience of cancer had brought significant changes, some perhaps forever. To my amazement, some of the changes had proven to be good. After years of seeking a means to witness for Christ, cancer had become the vehicle by which I could most easily do so. I thought now of Joni Erickson Tada, whose diving accident as a teen left her a quadriplegic. In her book, *Secret Strength*, Joni proclaimed that "God's power shows up best in weak people."

I recalled that the Apostle Paul had written similar words regarding a physical ailment that plagued him. "My grace is all you need," he said in his second letter to the Corinthians (12:9), "for my power is strongest when you are weak." I understood this claim better now, for the same seemed true for me. As others looked at my weakened, fatigued body, I'd had the privilege of showing them God's power within.

The family room was blissfully serene. I slid lower on the couch and watched red and yellow flames dance in the fireplace, snaking in and around the blazing logs. A pile of hot, glowing ashes had formed beneath the metal grate. The aroma of burning wood filled the air. I relaxed contentedly beside Bob as memories from a recent Sunday sermon spiraled upward from the glowing cinders. "We are not victims," the minister had said, "but conquerors." He, too, had battled cancer and overcome.

The late hour had an ethereal feeling, a magical dreaminess that was hard to define. I knew the past year had changed my life. My faith in God had grown enormously, and the highest dreams I'd held for Bob and me had been realized. Like the beautiful roses he had placed in my car, our love had blossomed, each day more joyful than the last.

The fire crackled invitingly. Bob's arm slid lovingly behind my back. *Who needs a party to celebrate?* I thought. What could be better than this?

I slid closer to my husband. With God's help and powerful medicines, it appeared we had conquered cancer. Tears of gratitude welled in my eyes. In the flickering flames, I could almost see an outline of the beautiful dove of summer. Words that had carried me this far flashed through my thoughts. "I will trust in Him, and not be afraid."

The television chimes rang out the midnight hour. Bob turned to kiss me. A new year had begun.

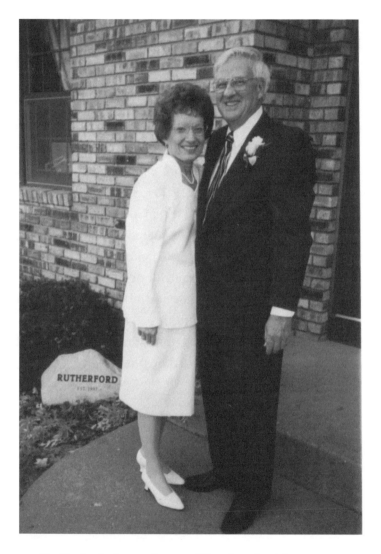

Jim Rutherford came into my life at just the right moment.
October 4, 1997.

Afterword

"For God so loved the world, that He gave His only begotten son, that whosoever believeth in Him should not perish, but have everlasting life."

John 3:16 KJV

In any worst-case scenario, the series of events that occurred during the writing of this book could never have been imagined.

On February 9, 1992—minutes after our weekly Sunday evening tennis hour with Sandy and Page—Bob, at age 55, suffered a massive heart attack in the club locker room and died. Three weeks earlier a series of tests had revealed a strong heart and steady rhythm; Bob and I had praised God for the good report. Then, with little warning, he was gone. I didn't get to kiss him goodbye.

For years I sought reasons for this unexplained loss and the resulting heartache in my life. Why, after the best years of our life together, should I be forced into this lonely life without Bob? At age 54, I was too young to be alone!

As with breast cancer, I realized, at last, the answers I sought were unknowable. I understood too—as God faithfully proved—that His love would carry me through this great sorrow.

In 1995 (three years later—after a lengthy battle with prostate cancer) my loving father, Lowell Woodall, joined Bob and God in eternity.

Shortly before his death, my twin, Deliece, was diagnosed with ovarian cancer. My mind would not allow me to accept the seriousness of her illness. Still, I traveled often to Villa Grove to be with her during repeated hospitalizations. She fought valiantly, but on March 26, 1997, she, too, passed from my life.

Without the presence of the Holy Spirit, faithful friends, loving, caring children and their spouses (Terry and Anne have since married) and five precious grandchildren, I could never have endured so much grief.

Happy memories helped sustain me. What I wrote of the loving relationship between Bob and me was a mere prelude to five glorious years. Ironically, only two months before Bob's death, I retired from my secretarial position at Moline High School. Our dreams of retirement years were to be unfulfilled, but in 1988, the year after breast cancer, we delighted in a memorable trip to Europe.

Today, after thirteen years, I have had no further encounters with cancer. My hair grew back curlier than before, and everyone who knows me understands about hot flashes; they never went away.

In the difficult years since Bob's death, writing has given me a much-needed focus. Often I would lose myself at the computer, groping for the right word or phrase, reliving the past, releasing my pain through the printed word.

Life is complex, to say the least, and filled with surprise. I've often marveled to think I was the one for whom many feared death, but I have survived while others dear to me have passed on. In the subsequent desolate days I've learned more than ever that out of adversity one develops inner strength and—from my experience—purer knowledge of God, greater compassion for others, truer patience concerning the future and genuine acceptance of life. I've also learned much about God's grace, and how very much He loves me.

To my absolute amazement, and when I least expected it, God proved that love once again by bringing a wonderful new man into my life. I'd hoped and prayed often for a new partner, but God's choice for me exceeded my fondest hopes and dreams. On October 4, 1997, surrounded by our six married children and twelve grandchildren, James Rutherford and I were married in First United Methodist Church, Moline, Illinois. Candles of remembrance were lit to honor Bob, Deliece, and Jim's wife, Helen, who died after an extended illness the previous year.

So, a new, exciting life has begun for us. If God can take all the heartaches of our lives and turn them into incredible joy, imagine what He can do for you!

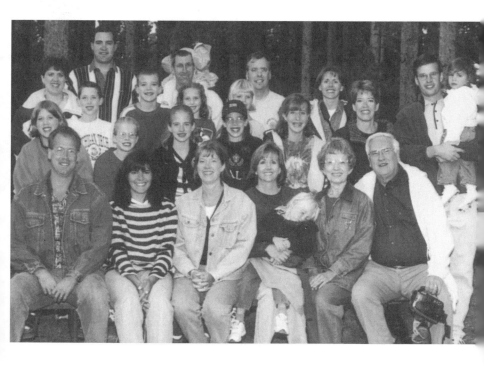

A gathering of the Hacketts and Rutherfords in Colorado, 1999.